MW00335088

Occupational Therapy Practice Guidelines for

Early Childhood: Birth Through 5 Years

Gloria Frolek Clark, PhD, OTR/L, BCP, FAOTA
Private Practice
Adel, IA

Karrie Kingsley, OTD, OTR/L
Assistant Professor of Clinical Occupational Therapy
University of Southern California
Division of Occupational Science and Occupational Therapy
Los Angeles

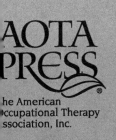

AOTA PRESS

he American
ccupational Therapy
ssociation, Inc.

AOTA Centennial Vision

We envision that occupational therapy is a powerful, widely recognized, science-driven, and evidence-based profession with a globally connected and diverse workforce meeting society's occupational needs.

AOTA Vision Statement

The American Occupational Therapy Association advances occupational therapy as the pre-eminent profession in promoting the health, productivity, and quality of life of individuals and society through the therapeutic application of occupation.

AOTA Mission Statement

The American Occupational Therapy Association advances the quality, availability, use, and support of occupational therapy through standard-setting, advocacy, education, and research on behalf of its members and the public.

AOTA Staff

Frederick P. Somers, *Executive Director*
Christopher M. Bluhm, *Chief Operating Officer*

Chris Davis, *Director, AOTA Press*
Ashley Hofmann, *Development/Production Editor*
Victoria Davis, *Digital/Production Editor*

Beth Ledford, *Director, Marketing*
Amanda Fogle, *Marketing Specialist*
Jennifer Folden, *Marketing Specialist*

The American Occupational Therapy Association, Inc.
4720 Montgomery Lane
Bethesda, MD 20814
301-652-AOTA (2682)
TDD: 800-377-8555
Fax: 301-652-7711
www.aota.org

To order: 1-877-404-AOTA (2682)

Disclaimers

This publication is designed to provide accurate and authoritative information in regard to the subject matter covered. It is sold or distributed with the understanding that the publisher is not engaged in rendering legal, accounting, or other professional service. If legal advice or other expert assistance is required, the services of a competent professional person should be sought.
—*From the Declaration of Principles jointly adopted by the American Bar Association and a Committee of Publishers and Associations*

It is the objective of the American Occupational Therapy Association to be a forum for free expression and interchange of ideas. The opinions expressed by the contributors to this work are their own and not necessarily those of the American Occupational Therapy Association.

ISBN-13: 978-1-56900-343-5
Library of Congress Control Number: 2013937576

Cover design by Jennifer Folden
Composition by Maryland Composition, Laurel, MD
Printing by Automated Graphics Systems, White Plains, MD

Contents

Summary and Implications for Occupational Therapy Practice

Acknowledgments

The series editor for this Practice Guideline is

Deborah Lieberman, MHSA, OTR/L, FAOTA
Director, Evidence-Based Practice
Staff Liaison to the Commission on Practice
American Occupational Therapy Association
Bethesda, MD

The issue editor for this Practice Guideline is

Marian Arbesman, PhD, OTR/L
President, ArbesIdeas, Inc.
Consultant, AOTA Evidence-Based Practice Project
Clinical Assistant Professor, Department of
  Rehabilitation Science
State University of New York at Buffalo

The authors acknowledge the following individuals
for their contribution to the evidence-based literature review:

Meghan E. Barnett, OTR
Meredith A. Carr, OTR
Jane Case-Smith, EdD, OTR, BCP, FAOTA
Breanne L. Hinkle, OTR
Tsu-Hsin Howe, PhD, OTR
Diane H. Kellegrew, PhD, OTR/L
Jennifer L. Kluever, OTR
Zoe Mailloux, OTD, OTR/L, FAOTA
Nicole M. Rowold, OTR
Theresa L. Schlabach, PhD, OTR/L, BCP
Tien-Ni Wang, PhD, OT
Amanda L. Wheelock, OTR

The authors acknowledge and thank the following
individuals for their participation in the content
review and development of this publication:

Jane Case-Smith, EdD, OTR, BCP, FAOTA
Dottie Handley-More, MS, OTR/L
Tsu-Hsin Howe, PhD, OTR
Zoe Mailloux, OTD, OTR/L, FAOTA
Theresa L. Schlabach, PhD, OTR/L, BCP
Tim Nanof, MSW
Sandra Schefkind, MS, OTR/L
V. Judith Thomas, MGA
Madalene Palmer

Note. The authors of this Practice Guideline have
signed a Conflict of Interest statement indicating
that they have no conflicts that would bear on this
work.

Introduction

Occupational therapists and occupational therapy assistants work with families and other caregivers to support and enhance young children's ability to engage in occupations appropriate to their age (e.g., sleep, play, eating). *Early childhood* is a term used to describe young children, generally birth through 5 years, and is used by the American Occupational Therapy Association (AOTA; Jackson, 2007) as well as other professional organizations such as the American Academy of Pediatrics, American Academy of Pediatric Dentistry, Council for Exceptional Children, and National Association for the Education of Young Children. This publication addresses occupational therapy practice that focuses on children from birth through age 5 years and includes early intervention and preschool practice. This is a critical time not only to educate the children but also to foster their ability to participate fully through all the years of their lives (Chandler, 2010).

Purpose and Use of This Publication

Practice guidelines have been widely developed in response to the health care reform movement in the United States. Such guidelines can be useful tools for improving the quality of health care, enhancing consumer satisfaction, promoting appropriate use of services, and reducing costs. AOTA, which represents the interests of 140,000 occupational therapists, occupational therapy assistants (see Appendix A), and students of occupational therapy, is committed to providing information through

relevant practice guidelines and other resources to support decision making that promotes high-quality health care and wellness and educational systems that are affordable and accessible to all. Readers should refer to current AOTA resources and those related to early childhood in the children and youth section of AOTA's website.

Using an evidence-based perspective and key concepts from the *Occupational Therapy Practice Framework: Domain and Process* (AOTA, 2008), this guideline provides an overview of the occupational therapy process for children from birth through age 5 years. It defines the occupational therapy domain, process, and intervention that occur within the boundaries of acceptable practice. This guideline does not discuss all possible methods of care, and although it does recommend some specific methods in practice, the occupational therapist makes the ultimate judgment regarding the appropriateness of a given procedure in light of a specific client's circumstances and needs.

It is the intention of AOTA, through this publication, to help occupational therapy practitioners, as well as individuals who manage, reimburse, or set policy regarding occupational therapy services, understand the contribution of occupational therapy in evaluating and serving children from birth through age 5. This guideline also can serve as a resource for parents, school administrators, educators, and other early childhood staff.

This document may be used in any of the following ways:

- To assist occupational therapists and occupational therapy assistants in communicating about their services to external audiences

- To assist other health care practitioners, teachers, and program administrators in determining whether referral for occupational therapy services would be appropriate
- To assist third-party payers in understanding the medical necessity and the therapeutic need for occupational therapy services for children birth through 5
- To assist health and education planning teams in determining the developmental and educational need for occupational therapy services
- To assist legislators, third-party payers, and administrators in understanding the professional education, training, and skills of occupational therapists and occupational therapy assistants
- To assist program developers, administrators, legislators, and third-party payers in understanding the scope of occupational therapy services
- To assist program evaluators and policy analysts in determining outcome measures for analyzing the effectiveness of occupational therapy intervention
- To assist policy, education, and health care benefit analysts in understanding the appropriateness of occupational therapy services for children from birth through 5
- To assist occupational therapy educators in designing appropriate curricula that incorporate the role of occupational therapy with children from birth through 5.

The introductory paragraphs of this guideline include a brief discussion of the domain and process of occupational therapy. Next, an overview of early childhood is provided. After this overview, a detailed discussion of the occupational therapy process for children from birth through 5 is presented. Intervention and evidence-based practice for early childhood are then provided, including a summary of the results of an evidence-based literature review for best practices early childhood occupational therapy. Implications for practice, education, research, and policy are discussed, followed by appendixes containing additional information for occupational therapists and occupational therapy assistants relating to early childhood practice, coding for intervention and evaluations, funding sources affecting early childhood settings, and methodologies used in the evidence-based literature review.

Domain and Process of Occupational Therapy

Occupational therapy practitioners'[1] expertise lies in their knowledge of occupation and how engaging in occupations can be used to improve human performance and ameliorate the effects of disease and disability (AOTA, 2008).

In 2002, the AOTA Representative Assembly adopted the *Occupational Therapy Practice Framework: Domain and Process*. Informed by the previous *Uniform Terminology for Occupational Therapy* (AOTA, 1979, 1989, 1994) and the World Health Organization's *International Classifcation of Functioning, Disability and Health* (WHO, 2001), the *Framework* outlines the profession's domain and the process of service delivery within this domain. In 2008, the *Framework* was updated as part of the standard 5-year review cycle (AOTA, 2008). The revisions included in the second edition focused on refining the document and updating it to reflect language and concepts relevant to current and emerging occupational therapy practice.

Domain

A profession's *domain* articulates its members' sphere of knowledge, societal contribution, and

---

[1]When the term *occupational therapy practitioner* is used in this document, it refers to both occupational therapists and occupational therapy assistants (AOTA, 2006).

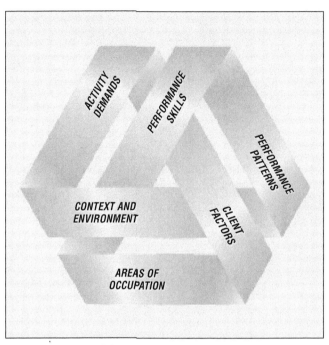

Figure 1. Occupational therapy's domain.

Reprinted from "Occupational Therapy Practice Framework: Domain and Process" (2nd ed., p. 627), by American Occupational Therapy Association, 2008, *American Journal of Occupational Theraphy, 62,* 625–683. Used with permission.

intellectual or scientific activity. The occupational therapy profession's domain centers on helping clients participate in daily life activities. The broad term that the profession uses to describe daily life activities is *occupation* (AOTA, 2008). Young children do not exist alone but are part of a relationship (Holloway, 1998; Holloway & Chandler, 2010; Winnicott, 1964). Occupational therapy practitioners recognize the relationships within the child's context and collaborate with these individuals to enhance the child's development. In this guideline,

the term *client*[2] includes the child as well as families, teachers, caregivers, and relevant others in the child's life.

As outlined in the *Framework*, occupational therapists and occupational therapy assistants[3] work collaboratively with clients to support health and participation through engagement in occupation (see Figure 1). This overarching mission circumscribes the profession's domain and emphasizes the important ways in which environmental and life circumstances influence the manner in

[2]For the purpose of this Practice Guideline, *client* includes the child and family/caregiver. If child is in preschool, the "client" may include the child, family, and teacher.

[3]*Occupational therapists* are responsible for all aspects of occupational therapy service delivery and are accountable for the safety and effectiveness of the occupational therapy service delivery process. *Occupational therapy assistants* deliver occupational therapy services under the supervision of, and in partnership with, an occupational therapist (AOTA, 2009)

AREAS OF OCCUPATION	CLIENT FACTORS	PERFORMANCE SKILLS	PERFORMANCE PATTERNS	CONTEXT AND ENVIRONMENT	ACTIVITY DEMANDS
Activities of Daily Living (ADL)* Instrumental Activities of Daily Living (IADL) Rest and Sleep Education Work Play Leisure Social Participation *Also referred to as *basic activities of daily living (BADL)* or *personal activities of daily living (PADL)*.	Values, Beliefs, and Spirituality Body Functions Body Structures	Sensory Perceptual Skills Motor and Praxis Skills Emotional Regulation Skills Cognitive Skills Communication and Social Skills	Habits Routines Roles Rituals	Cultural Personal Physical Social Temporal Virtual	Objects Used and Their Properties Space Demands Social Demands Sequencing and Timing Required Actions Required Body Functions Required Body Structures

Figure 2. Aspects of occupational therapy's domain.

Reprinted from "Occupational Therapy Practice Framework: Domain and Process" (2nd ed., p. 628), by American Occupational Therapy Association, 2008, *American Journal of Occupational Therapy, 62,* 625–683. Used with permission.

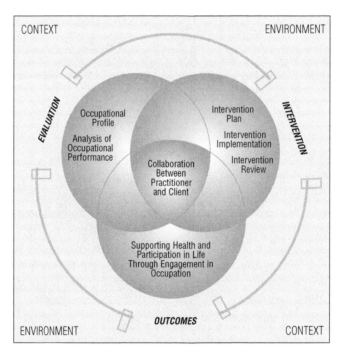

Figure 3. Occupational therapy's process of service delivery as applied within the profession's domain.

Reprinted from "Occupational Therapy Practice Framework: Domain and Process" (2nd ed., p. 627), by American Occupational Therapy Association, 2008, *American Journal of Occupational Therapy, 62,* 625–683. Used with permission.

which people carry out their occupations. Key aspects of the domain of occupational therapy are listed in Figure 2.

Process

Many professions use the process of evaluating, intervening, and targeting outcomes that is outlined in the *Framework*. Occupational therapy's application of this process is made unique, however, by its focus on occupation (see Figure 3). The process of occupational therapy service delivery typically begins with the *occupational profile*—an assessment of the client's occupational needs, problems, and concerns—and the *analysis of occupational performance*, which includes the skills, patterns, contexts, activity demands, and client factors that contribute

to or impede the client's satisfaction with his or her ability to engage in valued daily life activities. Therapists plan and implement intervention using a variety of approaches and methods in which occupation is both the means and the end (Gray, 1998; Trombly, 1995).

Occupational therapists continually assess the effectiveness of the intervention they provide and the client's progress toward targeted outcomes. Ongoing *intervention reviews* inform decisions to continue or discontinue intervention and to make referrals to other agencies or professionals. Therapists select outcome measures that are valid, reliable, and appropriately sensitive to the client's occupational performance, adaptation, health and wellness, prevention, quality of life, role competence, self-advocacy, and occupational justice.

Overview of Early Childhood

Prevalence of Common Disabilities

Currently, 20% of children in the United States under the age of 6 live in poverty (Karoly, Kilburn, & Cannon, 2005); however, in female-headed households, this percentage increases to 53. Children in poverty have fewer opportunities than their peers in access to resources (e.g., quality child care, health facilities) that are important for child development (Karoly et al., 2005). From 1997 to 2008, the number of children ages 3 through 17 years in the United States with developmental disabilities increased by 17.1% (Boyle et al., 2011). Currently, the prevalence of any developmental disability is 13.87%, or about 1 out of every 6 children (Boyle et al., 2011). This study also found boys had twice the frequency of any developmental disabilities as girls and that children whose family's income was below the poverty level had a higher prevalence of developmental disabilities. These delays may be mild to severe and include motor, social, cognitive, communication, and adaptive skills (e.g., eating).

Early identification of development delays is critical. The Centers for Disease Control and Prevention (CDC, n.d.) reported that more than 50% of parents do not know the warning signs of developmental delays, including autism. Occupational therapists, as the frontline providers in naturally occurring activities (e.g., play, feeding, social interactions), often recognize early signs of delay, and thus they need to screen children for these delays. The use of standardized screening measures (e.g., Modified Checklist for Autism in Toddlers [Robins, Fein, & Barton, 1999], Ages & Stages Questionnaires [Squires & Bricker, 2009]) is important to providing reliable and valid data for further decision making. Referral for further testing and evaluation may be appropriate. Early identification leads to earlier services, which have been shown to produce a positive effect on a child's development, academic achievement (Casto & Mastropieri, 1986; Innocenti & White, 1993), and prosocial behavior and employment (Karoly et al., 2005).

During the 2010 fiscal year, only 2.82% of the children in the United States between the ages of 0 and 2 years (approximately 343,821 children) received services under the Individuals with Disabilities Education Act of 1997 (IDEA; Pub. L. 108–446) Part C, Infant and Toddler Program (National Early Childhood Technical Assistance Center, 2012). IDEA requires participating states to provide early intervention services for infants and toddlers who have a diagnosed mental or physical condition or have documented developmental delays and their families (IDEA, 2004). In addition, an estimated 5.94% of preschoolers in the United States receive services and supports under IDEA Part B, with 2.2% in the Developmental Delay category (Office of Special Education Programs, 2010).

Prematurity

A National Vital Statistics Report estimated that 12% of babies (more than 500,000/year) born in the United States during 2010 were born before

37 weeks of pregnancy (Hamilton, Martin, & Ventura, 2011). Prematurity increases the risk of health complications (e.g., respiration distress, jaundice, seizures, apnea, feeding difficulties) and disabilities (e.g., intellectual or learning disabilities, behavioral problems, cerebral palsy [CP], vision and hearing loss, respiratory complications). Studies indicate that children who are born premature have an increased risk of autism (Limperopoulos et al., 2008; Schendel & Bhasin, 2008) and adult health problems (e.g., heart disease, diabetes, high blood pressure; Hovi et al., 2007).

Autism Spectrum Disorders

The Autism and Developmental Disabilities Monitoring Network, established by the CDC, now estimates that the prevalence of autism spectrum disorders (ASD) is 1 in 88 children (1 in 54 boys and 1 in 252 girls; CDC, 2012a). Symptoms of ASD often are present before age 3 years and include difficulties in cognitive functioning, learning, attention, and sensory processing (Yeargin-Allsopp et al., 2003). The Autism and Developmental Disabilities Monitoring Network data indicated that 62% of children with ASD do not have an intellectual disability and that there is an 83% co-occurrence with non-ASD developmental diagnoses (e.g., genetic, neurologic, chromosomal, psychiatric). The average medical costs for Medicaid-enrolled children with ASD were about 6 times higher than for children without ASD (Peacock, Amendah, Ouyang, & Grosse, 2012).

Feeding Disorders

Feeding disorders are common in children developing typically. An estimated 25% to 45% of children have feeding problems (Linscheid, 1992; Manikam & Perman, 2000); this number rises to 80% when children with developmental delays are included (Manikam & Perman, 2000). Feeding problems may include lack of self-feeding, food refusal, lack of appetite, and aggression at mealtimes (Berlin, Davies, Silverman, & Rudolph, 2009). Feeding disorders may include gastrointestinal disorders, abnormal feeding patterns, and difficulty with food intake. They can lead to growth failure, susceptibility to chronic illness, and, sometimes, death (Manikam & Perman, 2000).

Obesity

Obesity is also a significant medical condition in the United States. Anderson and Whitaker (2009) estimated the obesity prevalence among 4- to 5-year-olds to be 18.4%. The consequences of childhood obesity include health risks such as high blood pressure, high cholesterol, increased risk of Type 2 diabetes, sleep apnea, asthma, joint problems, fatty liver disease, gastroesophageal reflux, and social and psychological problems (CDC, 2012a).

Family-Centered Services and Partnerships With Families

Given the dependence of young children on adults, families and caregivers play a critical role in their child's health and development. Developing positive partnerships with the family or caregivers is essential for professionals. The role of parents as decision makers and partners in setting goals for their children was solidified in 1975 with the adoption of Public Law 94–142 (the Education for All Handicapped Children Act of 1975) and continue to be emphasized in IDEA (2004). Turnbull, Turnbull, Erwin, Soodak, and Shogren (2011) provided five characteristics of family-centeredness in services:
1. Professionals ensure families are the ultimate decision makers;
2. Services build on families' strengths;
3. The services and support focus on the family as the unit, not the child;

4. Services emphasize a positive relationship with the family/caregiver; and
5. Services are individualized to families.

Although many early childhood professionals embrace the philosophy of family-centered service, they do not implement the elements of family-centered services in practice (Dunst, 2002).

Funding Sources That Affect Occupational Therapy Services

Several federal laws influence occupational therapy practice. AOTA (2011) reviewed the more common laws related to early childhood (see Table 1).

Table 1. Federal Laws and Their Influence on Occupational Therapy Services

Law	Influence on Occupational Therapy Services
Individuals with Disabilities Education Improvement Act (IDEA), Pub. L. 108–446	Federal legislation that specifically includes occupational therapy as a related service for eligible students with disabilities, ages 3–21 years, to benefit from special education (Part B) or as a primary service for infants and toddlers who are experiencing developmental delays (Part C).
Elementary and Secondary Education Act (ESEA) Amendments, No Child Left Behind Act, Pub. L. 107–110	Federal legislation that requires public schools to raise the educational achievement of all students, particularly those from disadvantaged backgrounds, students with disabilities, and those with limited English proficiency, and that states establish high standards for teaching and student learning. Though not specifically mentioned in the statute, occupational therapy is generally considered to be a pupil service under ESEA.
Improving Head Start for School Readiness Act of 2007, Pub. L. 110–134	Federal program that provides comprehensive child development services to economically disadvantaged children (ages birth–5 years) and their families, including children with disabilities. Early Head Start serves children up to 3 years of age. Occupational therapy may be provided in these settings under the Head Start requirements or under IDEA.
Section 504 of the Rehabilitation Act of 1973, as amended, 29 U.S.C. 794; Americans with Disabilities Act (ADA, as amended); Americans with Disabilities Act Amendments of 2008 (ADAAA), Pub. L. 110–325	Civil rights statutes that prohibit discrimination on the basis of disability by programs receiving federal funds (Section 504) and by services and activities of state and local government (ADA and ADAAA). *Disability* here is defined more broadly than in IDEA. Children and youth who are not eligible for IDEA may be eligible for services under Section 504 or the ADA, such as for environmental adaptations and other reasonable accommodations, to help them access and succeed in the learning environment. Each state or local education agency determines eligibility procedures for children and youth served under Section 504 or the ADA.
Title XIX of the Social Security Act of 1965, as amended; Medicaid, Pub. L. 89–97	Federal–state match program that provides medical and health services for low-income children and adults. Occupational therapy is an optional service under the state plan but mandatory for children and youth under the Early Periodic Screening, Diagnosis and Treatment (EPSDT) services mandate.
Assistive Technology Act of 2004, Pub. L. 108–364, as amended	Federal program that promotes access to assistive technology for persons with disabilities so that they can more fully participate in education, employment, and daily activities.
U.S. Department of Agriculture Food and Nutrition Service (2001)	National school breakfast and lunch programs are required to provide food substitutions and modifications of school meals for students whose disabilities restrict their diets, as determined by a doctor.

Note. From "Occupational Therapy Services in Early Childhood and School-Based Settings," by American Occupational Therapy Association, 2011, *American Journal of Occupational Therapy, 65*(6 Suppl.), p. S47. Copyright © 2011 by the American Occupational Therapy Association. Adapted with permission.

Under some of these laws—for example, IDEA, Medicaid, and Head Start—states may receive funding for services, such as occupational therapy, for children who meet state or federal eligibility requirements. Other laws, such as Section 504 of the Rehabilitation Act of 1973, as amended (29 U.S.C. 794) and the Americans with Disabilities Act of 1990 (Pub. L. 101–336), do not provide additional funding; however, school districts are required to comply with the laws if they receive any federal funds. Occupational therapists may be members of the building's Section 504 team and, in some states, provide services to eligible children.

Emerging education initiatives, such as response to intervention (RtI), promote occupational therapy services to general education or community preschool staff, including professional development for staff and instructional suggestions for at-risk children.[4] Legislation such as Early Head Start, the Child Abuse and Prevention Treatment Act, and the Combating Autism Act of 2006 have increased the role of occupational therapists in the initial evaluation and program planning for young children.

If services are medically necessary, occupational therapy services may be funded through private insurance, Medicaid and waiver programs, or private pay. The number of treatments and coverage provided by insurance companies varies by policy, even within an insurance company. State Medicaid programs include Early and Periodic Screening, Diagnostic, and Treatment (EPSDT) and waiver programs that may be used to cover services. Private pay by the family is also an option.

Settings for Occupational Therapy Services

Occupational therapy practitioners provide necessary services to support children's health and participation in life through engagement in occupation across many environments, settings, and programs. During the early childhood years, these settings may include the home, preschool, community locations, and medical or clinic environments. Community settings could include locations where the family and child engage in their daily activities, such as the child's day care, parks where the child plays, grocery stores, and libraries.

The environment and funding may influence the focus of the occupational therapy services. For example, under IDEA Part C, services are required to be provided in the natural environment, such as home or community settings, to the maximum extent appropriate [§303.13(1)(8)]. The *natural environment* includes settings that are typical for peers without a disability (§303.26). Teams make the final decision regarding placement; however, the current Part C federal regulations' analysis of comments and changes section related to natural environments states that a natural environment does not includes a clinic, hospital, or service provider's office, and justification is necessary if services are provided in such environments (IDEA Early Intervention Program for Infants and Toddlers with Disabilities, 34 CFR Part 303, 2011).

Depending on the needs of the child and the funding sources, children could be receiving occupational therapy services in different environments from different therapists. For example, an infant with multiple medical needs (e.g., feeding tube, tracheotomy, hypertonia) may receive weekly occupational therapy services as an outpatient at the hospital with the goal of safe oral feeding. Through the early intervention program, an occupational therapy practitioner may be providing weekly services to the infant and his or her family to meet the child/family outcomes related to developing play and motor skills, developing the family's capacity to care for the infant's self-care and positioning needs, and following the oral/feeding home program from the hospital. Collaboration and communication among these professionals are critical for a smooth continuum of care for the child and family.

---

[4]Occupational therapy practitioners should refer to their state practice acts to identify professional activities allowed under screening.

Occupational Therapy Process for Children Birth Through 5 Years

Overview

The process of occupational therapy for young children (and their families, caregivers, and teachers) includes evaluation, intervention, and outcome planning to enhance the child's occupational performance, adaptation, health and wellness, participation in the community, quality of life, role competence, and self-advocacy (AOTA, 2008). The occupational therapy process aims to identify the individual's areas of strengths and needs related to engagement and participation in occupations and activities and includes collaboration and various team models to achieve these goals.

Evaluation

Services may be initiated when an individual client demonstrates functional difficulties that impede engagement in occupations and participation in everyday life. The evaluation includes gathering, interpreting, and synthesizing information relevant to the client's past and current occupational engagement and performance as well as exploring client's desired future participation.

Intervention

Occupational therapy intervention is individually designed and is aimed at improving the client's desired and expected occupational engagement and participation through implementation of strategies and procedures directed at the client, the activity, and the environment (context; AOTA, 2008, 2011; Carrasco et al., 2007). When developing an inter-

vention plan, the occupational therapist always considers the dynamic nature of the context in which the client is expected to perform the activity.

Outcomes Planning

The occupational therapy process also includes monitoring the client's response to the intervention, reevaluating and modifying the intervention plan, and measuring intervention success through outcomes that are relevant and meaningful to the individual. The *Framework* (AOTA, 2008) uses a *client-centered approach* adapted from Dunn (2000), defined as "an orientation that honors the desires and priorities of clients in designing and implementing interventions" (p. 670). Occupational therapy practitioners working in early intervention (IDEA Part C) use a family-centered model, in which the family members are active participants and ultimate decision makers in supports and services (Pletcher & McBride, 2000; Polichino, Clark, Swinth, & Muhlenhaupt, 2007; Turnbull et al., 2011). When working with preschoolers, occupational therapy practitioners may focus on the child but also include parents, educational staff, and the school system (AOTA, 2011; Polichino et al., 2007). The occupational therapy process considers the dynamic interaction of the client and the internal neurophysiological and external physical, social, and cultural contexts of function.

Clinical reasoning is used throughout the process. Occupational therapy services should be dynamic and interactive. Engagement in occupations is typically used as both the method and desired outcome of the process (Trombly, 1995).

Collaboration

Collaborative relationships are developed between occupational therapists and their clients in order to understand their experiences and intervention outcomes (AOTA, 2008; Clark, 2010). As occupational therapy practitioners work with young children, they may collaborate with individuals (e.g., the child, family, caregivers, teachers, physicians, other health care providers) and work with organizations (e.g., community preschools; Head Start; Women, Infants, and Children programs) and populations (e.g., programs for children residing in homeless shelters and foster care).

Team Models

Successful team interaction is essential for effective intervention services (Bose & Hinojosa, 2008; Turnbull et al., 2011). Regardless of the setting, occupational therapy practitioners are typically members of a team. The three team models commonly used in early childhood services include the (a) multidisciplinary, (b) interdisciplinary, and (c) transdisciplinary team approach.

Members of the *multidisciplinary* model evaluate the child separately and select treatment goals and approaches based on their professional findings. Parallel provision of services is common in medical settings (Carrasco et al., 2007). *Interdisciplinary teams* are commonly used in school-based practices in which team members complete evaluations, either alone or together, and then meet as a group to collaboratively plan and develop goals (Carrasco et al., 2007; Foss, 2010). Although each discipline provides services separately, team members are committed to frequent communication and collaboration to coordinate a comprehensive plan of services and maximize the child's outcomes.

Team members in a *transdisciplinary* team model do not follow traditional disciplinary boundaries but instead share the responsibility of the child's initial evaluation and establish goals with the families. Typically, any team member whose expertise fits with the child and family's needs provides the service.[5] Sometimes co-service providers are used when the child has multiple needs that are best addressed by different professionals. Other team members provide consultation to share skills and knowledge with the primary team member (Case-Smith, 2005). Many early intervention teams use the transdisciplinary model (Foss, 2010) when working in homes and community settings.

The primary service provider (PSP) uses traditional intervention model (e.g., deficit focused, expert driven) or coaching model (i.e., interactive process that promotes family's ability to support child's participation; Holloway & Chandler, 2010). A coaching model is supported by early childhood literature (S. K. Campbell, 1997; Dinnebeil, McInerney, Roth, & Ramasway, 2001; Hanft & Pilkington, 2000; Hanft, Rush, & Shelden, 2004). Rush and Shelden (2011) described *coaching* "as an evidence-based practice . . . that is used intentionally to partner with parents in order to build their capacity to identify priories and achieve their desired outcomes" (p. 22). The coaching process generally requires joint planning with the family or caregiver, observation of the child, action or practice opportunities, reflection following the practice opportunities to generate alternative actions, and feedback from the coach.

---

[5]This model allows that an occupational therapist could be the primary service provider (PSP) for some children while providing consultation to other PSPs and children. Occupational therapy practitioners should review their state licensure and proceed with caution if they are asked to provide services outside of their scope of practice.

Referrals and Requests for Services

The occupational therapy process is typically initiated by a referral from the family or caregiver, physician, or school personnel; however, IDEA 2004 requires specific procedures, which are discussed later in this section. The reason for referral often depends on the setting, age of the child, and funding source. Typically, occupational therapy services are requested when performance limitations are present (e.g., in movement, play, self-regulation, social interactions, fine motor function, self-care) or as part of a team evaluation.

A referral for an occupational therapy evaluation under IDEA Part C (infants and toddlers) or Part B (preschoolers and school-age children) must follow this federal law and regulations, individual state regulations, and comply with occupational therapy state practice acts. Informed written consent must be obtained from the parent before evaluations can be conducted. Under Part C (in most states, this would include children who are younger than 3 years old), the multidisciplinary evaluation must include the following areas: cognitive, physical (includes vision and hearing), communication, social or emotional, and adaptive development. An occupational therapist could be part of the diagnostic assessment team to determine eligibility, conduct an evaluation to determine the child's strengths and needs relative to occupational performance and daily life/daily activities in the domain of occupational therapy, and conduct the family assessment. In some situations an occupational therapy evaluation may not be needed initially, but the team may request one later later. State procedures should be followed to obtain parent consent for an occupational therapy evaluation.

Under IDEA Part B (i.e., children older than age 3 years), a request for an initial evaluation typically comes from the parent of a child, a state agency, or a local educational agency. Informed written consent from parents is necessary to conduct a full and individual initial evaluation to determine eligibility

for special education before special education instructional and related services (e.g., occupational therapy) are provided (§1414 [1]). However, if occupational therapy is not part of the initial evaluation process, and if a child is found eligible for special education, an occupational therapy evaluation to determine need for services may be conducted later, following state procedures to obtain parent consent.

Evaluation Considerations

In most cases, an occupational therapy evaluation is ultimately requested to document the child's strengths and weaknesses and to determine whether intervention by an occupational therapist is needed to assist the child in improving engagement in everyday life activities. Under IDEA Part C, occupational therapy services are provided to eligible children if "necessary to meet the unique needs of the child and family to achieve the results of outcomes identified" by the individualized family service plan (IFSP) team [§303.344(d)]. Evaluation should include the child's developmental skills as well as a family-directed assessment of their resources, priorities, and concerns necessary to build the family's capacity to care for their child's developmental needs.

Under Part B, occupational therapy services are provided when "required to assist a child with a disability to benefit from special education" (§300.34[a]). An occupational therapy evaluation should gather "relevant functional, developmental and academic information about the child" (§300.304[b][1]), performance in their curriculum or participation in appropriate activities (§300.304[b][1][ii]), and include multiple measures.

Evaluations have different purposes, so occupational therapists must know the intent of the referral (e.g., screening, diagnostic, or program planning) before gathering data (see Table 2). As members of educational or early intervention multidisciplinary teams, occupational therapists may participate in evaluations to determine a child's diagnosis

Table 2. Purposes of Evaluation in Early Childhood

Purpose	Answers What Question	Under IDEA	Medical Settings
Screening	Does this child need further evaluation by an occupational therapist?	*Under Part C (0–3 years):* Determine need for further evaluation. *Under Part B (3–21 years):* Provide support for general education instruction or for Child Find purposes.	Determine need for further evaluation.
Diagnostic (occupational therapists, as members of multidisciplinary teams, may participate in determining educational diagnosis or eligibility for services)	Is this child's performance typical or atypical to peers? What are the child's strengths? Needs?	Identify the child's strengths and needs to determine eligibility for early intervention or special education.	Identify the child's strengths and needs to determine need for medically necessary treatment (insurance coverage) or need for occupational therapy services (private funding).
Program planning with family and team	What outcomes and services are important for this child?	*Part C:* Identify the unique strengths and needs of the infant or toddler, develop outcomes, and identify services to meet these needs. *Part B:* Determine the educational needs, develop goals, and determine services appropriate to meet these needs.	Identify the child's strengths and needs and develop treatment plan with goals.
Program evaluation	Did we make a difference? What is the outcome of intervention? Has the child met the desired goal or outcome?	Ongoing assessment to determine progress toward outcomes. Determine ongoing eligibility for program and occupational therapy services (as appropriate).	Ongoing assessment to determine progress toward outcomes. Determine ongoing need for occupational therapy services.

Note. Modified from "Evaluation, Assessment, and Outcomes in Early Childhood," by G. F. Clark, 2010, in *Early Childhood: Occupational Therapy Services for Children Birth to Five* (p. 145), B. Chandler (Ed.), Bethesda, MD: AOTA Press. Copyright © 2011 by the American Occupational Therapy Association. Adapted with permission. IDEA = Individuals with Disabilities Education Act.

or eligibility for services (Clark, 2010; Clark & Coster, 1998; Stewart, 2010). As with occupational therapy evaluations conducted in a medical setting, therapists identify the client's occupational therapy treatment diagnosis.

The evaluation process should include measurement of the child's abilities in the various aspects of the domain of occupational therapy and use various methods to gather a comprehensive picture of the child's performance. These methods may include

- Reviewing records to gather information about medical history and diagnoses; developmental milestones; and, when appropriate, behaviors and performance in school;
- Interviewing family, caregivers, educational staff, and others who have relevant information;

- Observing the child during everyday life activities to gain insight into his or her ability abilities to organize, plan, and perform according to the demands of the task and within the environment; and
- Administering tests, including norm-referenced assessments, criterion-referenced assessments, and alternative or authentic assessments (data collected from the child's performance during his or her natural routines and activities, e.g., play-based assessments, structures child constructed with peers during free time in classroom; Clark, 2010; Losardo & Notari-Syverson, 2001).

Occupational therapists perform evaluations in collaboration with the client and target information specific to the desired outcomes. The two elements of the occupational therapy evaluation are (1) the occupational profile and (2) the analysis of occupational performance (AOTA, 2008).

Occupational therapists working with young children may use standardized and nonstandardized assessments that are specifically designed for this age group and population. Data collection may occur formally and informally during all interactions and observations of the child/family. Because children's behavior can vary from one setting to another or on the basis of individual perspectives, occupational therapists should use multiple methods to assess children (Achenbach, McConaughy, & Howell, 1987; McConaughy & Ritter, 2008; Sandall, Hemmeter, Smith, & McLean, 2005). Methods may include observation, interview, work samples, and formal and informal tools. IDEA requires the use of "variety of assessment tools and strategies" (§300.304[a][1]) and "not use any single measure or assessment as the sole criterion" (§300. 304[a][2]) for determining eligibility and appropriate educational program.

Role of the Family

One in four children with disabilities who resides with two parents lives in poverty (Cauthen & Fass, 2009). Wang (2005) found that households headed by a single mother were more likely to have a child with a disability than any other family type. The family is assumed to be the constant in the child's life and have the inherent strengths that serve as a foundation for the child's growth and development (Shelton & Stepanek, 1994).

Although the child is often considered the client, for young children the family also should be considered a client, because their care of the child is critical, and they have legal responsibility for the child. Encouraging and supporting their active participation in their child's life and development is important. Families have knowledge about the child and can contribute and assist during assessment and intervention planning (Clark, 2010; McLean & Crais, 2004).

The philosophy and practice of family-centered services provide the family a vital role in identifying the family/child's resources, concerns, priorities, and needs. "The ideal in family-centered services is for professionals to defer to the family in decision making regarding the nature and extent of services and supports for the young child and for other family members" (Turnbull et al., 2011, p. 105). The client-centered process used by occupational therapy practitioners honors the client's (e.g., child, family) desires and priorities and uses these during intervention planning and provision (AOTA, 2008). Regardless of the setting, collaborating with family is essential for understanding and building trust for an ongoing partnership.

Setting and Context

Occupational therapy practitioners work with young children in many settings (e.g., homes, hospitals, clinics, schools, child care centers, community) and with families and professionals (e.g., physicians, nurses, educators, speech–language pathologists, physical therapists, psychologists) and paraprofessionals (e.g., classroom assistants). The setting and funding source influence the focus and purpose of the evaluation (e.g., home, Part C early intervention, Part B preschool, Head Start, hospital).

For example, occupational therapists working in the neonatal intensive care unit (NICU) and with other medically fragile children provide services to enable basic life skills such as eating, grasping, or body movements.

Occupational therapists working in hospitals or clinics may focus on engagement and participation across multiple settings and contexts, including play skills, dressing, and social interactions with others. Working in a client's home or community settings, the occupational therapist may concentrate on enhancing the child's performance during the family routines and activities. Occupational therapists working in preschools address the child's performance and participation in academic and nonacademic activities (e.g., classroom work, social interactions, self-help, following rules).

Standardized vs. Nonstandardized Assessments

Occupational therapists use their knowledge of assessments and clinical judgment to decide which assessment methods should be selected for young children at a particular time. Standardized tools and norm-referenced assessments are useful for diagnostic purposes (e.g., determining eligibility or need for services) rather than program planning or monitoring ongoing progress (Clark, 2010). In early childhood and early intervention programs, the use of curriculum-based assessment is more common because it can be used for decision making from eligibility to progress monitoring (Macy, Bricker, & Squires, 2005; McLean, 2005; Neisworth & Bagnato, 2004). Occupational therapists use multiple methods to gather data regarding the child's occupational performance (Moyers & Dale, 2007).

Standardized assessments of various performance skills and client factors are routinely administered in hospitals and clinics to establish a baseline performance at the initiation of occupational therapy services and to provide objective and reliable measurement for quantitative documentation of clients' progress. Periodic reevaluations determine the client's progress and need for continued intervention.

Norm-referenced assessments are used primarily for diagnostic purposes, and *criterion-referenced assessments* are used to measure a child's mastery of skills. When using highly structured standardized assessments in contrived situations, occupational therapists verify the reliability of the results through family or caregiver interviews and observations during other situations.

Young children often do not perform on command and may be labeled "untestable" or score lower than their true abilities. Using evaluations that gather data during play or natural interactions provides more reliable and valid information in natural environments than contrived activities for assessment tools (Losardo & Notari-Syverson, 2001; Neisworth & Bagnato, 2004).

Alternative approaches, as outlined in Table 3, may provide more reliable information about the child's functional performance. *Embedded assessments*, such as those that are ecologically based or play-based, embed assessment within typical routines or interactions. *Authentic assessments* include actual products that were gathered as the child performed various tasks within the natural environment. For example, during block center, a photograph may be taken of the child's final construction. *Mediated assessments*, such as dynamic or curriculum-based assessments, can be used to identify the child's abilities and skills as well as help with program planning.

Occupational Profile

The occupational profile may be completed during the first visit or during ongoing visits as the client identifies why he or she is seeking serves, shares experiences, and identifies his or her priorities and outcomes. Information for the occupational profile is gathered through formal and informal interviews (see Box 1) with the client and significant

Table 3. Types of Early Childhood Assessment Methods

Method		Description	Examples
Norm-referenced assessment		Compares child's performance to a normative group of children; standardized	Battelle Developmental Inventory (Newborg, 2004); Bayley Scales of Infant Development (Bayley, 2005)
Criterion-referenced assessment		Indicates child's performance on specific skills	Learning Accomplishment Profile (Hardin & Peisner-Feinberg, 2004)
Alternative Approaches			
Embedded	Naturalistic	Embedded in child's routine, schedule, and environment	Ecologically based assessment of the child as she puts on clothing to go home (e.g., context, activity, materials, what peers can do, what target child can do)
	Focused	Adult-structured interactions to elicit child behaviors; activities may not necessarily be authentic	Play-based assessment: Request parents play a game with child in order for examiner to observe a child's ability to follow directions
Authentic	Performance	Actual products gathered from the child during tasks of the daily routine or specific activities for assessment	Videotapes, photographs, work samples
	Portfolio	Samples are collected using a clear process and evaluation criteria; child often active in gathering these work samples	Photographs of letters child formed during free time at preschool easel that are evaluated using a predetermined rubric
Mediated	Dynamic assessment	Test–teach–retest method of learning that supports predictions about child's response to interventions and future performance	Anecdotes of child's responses
	Curriculum-based assessment (CBA)	Specific type of criterion-referenced assessment that directly aligns with curricular content and provides programming suggestions	Assessment, Evaluation & Programming System (AEPS; Bricker & Waddell, 2002a, 2002b); Carolina Curriculum for Preschoolers with Special Needs (Johnson-Martin, Attermeier, & Hacker, 2004b); Creative Curriculum for Early Childhood (Dodge et al., 2010); Hawaii Early Learning Profile (HELP; Parks, 1992–2006)

Note. Modified from "Evaluation, Assessment, and Outcomes in Early Childhood," by G. F. Clark, 2010 in *Early Childhood: Occupational Therapy Services for Children Birth to Five* (p. 147), B. Chandler (Ed.), Bethesda, MD: AOTA Press. Copyright © 2011 by the American Occupational Therapy Association. Adapted with permission.

others (in the case of the very young or medically fragile child, the family, medical staff, caregiver, and/or teachers may provide input for the occupational profile). Conversations with the family help the occupational therapist gain a perspective of how the child spends his or her time; what activities the child wants or needs to do; and how the environment in which the child lives, plays, and attends school supports or hinders occupational engagement. Depending on the setting and child's needs, information is gathered during the initial contact with the family, child (when applicable), and significant others, and continues throughout the occupational therapy process.

Box 1. Sample Interview Questions Used for Developing Occupational Profile

1. Why are you seeking occupational therapy services for this child?
2. What is a typical day like for this child? (Describe routines and activities that typically occur; this information allows the therapist to understand the routines, valued activities, and the child's participation.)
3. What does this child enjoy doing during the day?
4. What do you think is going well at home? At preschool? At child care?
5. What do you see as concerns at home? At preschool? At child care?
6. Do you see the same difficulties in other locations?
7. Are there certain places or times when this child's performance seems to be better?
8. What activities have you tried to help this child's learning/development?
9. Tell me about the people who help you with this child's learning and growth. (Family: including the physician; this provides information about the family's resources.)
10. What do you think is interfering with this child's learning, growing, or participating?
11. What do you think needs to change?
12. What are your priorities for this child? How would you like occupational therapy to assist you and this child?

Note. Modified from "Evaluating Occupational Performance in Schools and Early Childhood Settings," by J. Polichino, G. F. Clark, Y. Swinth, and M. Muhlenhaupt, in *Occupational Therapy Services for Children and Youth Under IDEA* (pp. 31 and 40), by L. Jackson (Ed.), 2007, Bethesda, MD: AOTA Press. Copyright © 2007 by the American Occupational Therapy Association. Adapted with permission.

Developing the occupational profile involves the following steps:

- *Identify the client or clients.*
- *Determine why the client is seeking services.* Through interviews or checklists, the occupational therapist assists the client in identifying the current concerns relative to the areas of occupation and performance. This is a critical part of the evaluation and may be reviewed as the child develops new skills or the client changes the emphasis for intervention.
- *Identify the areas of occupation that are successful and the areas that are causing problems or risks.* On the basis of the client's current concerns, the occupational therapist identifies possible motor, cognitive, and behavioral impairments and environmental barriers and supports related to occupational performance.
- *Discuss significant aspects of the client's occupational history.* Significant aspects can include life experiences (e.g., medical interventions, family employment history, interests, previous patterns of engagement in occupations that provide meaning to the client's life). These experiences may shape how the child interacts with others during daily routines and occupations.
- *Determine the client's priorities and desired outcomes.* At various points in the provision of occupational therapy services, the occupational therapist and the client and/or family will discuss and prioritize outcomes so that the therapist's evaluation and intervention will match the client's/family's desired outcomes. Initially the client may be unable to share his or her hopes,

because of medical or developmental impairments; however, as the client progresses, the occupational therapist should review the priorities and desired outcomes with the client, adjusting these as necessary. The occupational therapist may need to refer the client to additional professionals to achieve some of the desired outcomes.

Analysis of Occupational Performance

The occupational therapist uses the information from the occupational profile to focus on the specific areas of occupation and the context and environment in which the child and family lives. On the basis of the practice setting; family priorities and concerns; and child's age, health, and medical needs, decisions are made about additional information that needs to be gathered before the child's occupational performance can be analyzed. To analyze occupational performance, the occupational therapist gathers information to understand the child's performance within his or her context (e.g., the hospital, home, community environments).

The *Framework* (AOTA, 2008) lists several steps the occupational therapist takes:

- *Synthesize information* gathered from the occupational profile and record review to focus on specific areas of occupation and contexts that need to be addressed.
- *Observe the child (and family, if possible)* as he or she performs the occupations in the natural or least restrictive environment (when possible) and document the effectiveness of the child's performance skills (e.g., motor and praxis, sensory–perceptual, cognitive, emotional regulation, communication and social) and performance patterns (e.g., habits, routines, rituals, roles) within the environment and interaction between the child, family, and others. When observing children in the hospital, therapists may use play, social interactions, or self-care activities to evaluate performance

skills and patterns. When observing children in preschools, observe the impact of the curriculum, instruction, and environment on the child's performance skills and patterns.

- *Select specific assessments and evaluation methods* that will identify and measure the factors related to the specific aspects of the domain that may be influencing the client's performance (and, in educational programs, assist teams in determining educational need; see Table 4 for examples of selected assessments).
- *Interpret the assessment data* to identify what supports or hinders performance in various environments and areas of occupations.
- *Develop or refine a hypothesis* regarding the child's performance.
- *Create goals for the occupational therapy intervention plan* in collaboration with the family and child that address their desired outcomes or achievements. If the child is hospitalized or has a medical diagnosis, collaboration with medical teams may be necessary to identify risks and precautions. Under IDEA, parents are included on the teams that develop the child's goals on the individualized education plan (IEP) and the child and family outcomes on the IFSP. As members of these teams, occupational therapists promote IEP goals and IFSP outcomes that promote health and participation in the child's occupations/activities.
- *Determine procedures to measure the outcomes* of the intervention.
- *Identify potential intervention approaches,* guided by best practice and the evidence, and share this information with the client.
- *Document the evaluation process and communicate the results* to family, the appropriate team members, and community agencies.

Occupational therapists evaluate performance in any of the areas of occupation by focusing on the activities and occupations that have been identified by family and caregivers and, when applicable, the child and school. Gathering data from multiple

Table 4. Selected Assessments of Occupational Performance for Early Childhood (Birth–5 Years)

Domain of Occupational Therapy	Sample Assessments Used by Occupational Therapists
Areas of Occupation	
• Activities of daily living • Instrumental activities of daily living • Rest and sleep • Education • Work • Play • Leisure • Social participation	• Asset-Based Context Matrix (Wilson et al., 2004) • Achenbach System of Empirically Based Assessment–Pre-School Module (Achenbach, 2009) • Adaptive Behavior Assessment System, 2nd ed. (Harrison & Oakland, 2003) • Behavior Assessment System for Children, 2nd ed. (Reynolds & Kamphaus, 2006) • Canadian Occupational Performance Measure (Law et al., 2005) • Children's Assessment of Participation and Environment and Preferences for Activities of Children (King et al., 2005) • Children's Engagement Questionnaire (McWilliam, 1991) • Choosing Outcomes and Accommodations for Children, 3rd ed. (Giangreco et al., 2011) • Knox Preschool Play Scale (Knox, 2008) • Miller Function and Participation Scales (Miller, 2006) • Pediatric Evaluation of Disability Inventory (Haley et al., 1992) • Paediatric Activity Card Sort (Mandich et al., 2004) • Play Preference Inventory (Wolfberg, 1995) • Preschool Activity Card Sort (Berg & LaVesser, 2006) • Scales of Independent Behavior–Revised (Bruininks et al., 1996) • School Version of the Assessment of Motor and Process Skills (Fisher et al., 2005) • Test of Playfulness (Skard & Bundy, 2008) • Transdiciplinary Play-Based Assessment, 2nd ed. (Linder, 2008) • Vineland Adaptive Behavior Scales, 2nd ed. (Sparrow et al., 2005) • WEE–FIM II (Uniform Data System for Medical Rehabilitation, 2003)
Performance Skills	
• Sensory–perceptual skills • Motor and praxis skills • Emotional regulation skills • Cognitive skills • Communication and social skills	• Adaptive Behavior Assessment System, 2nd ed. (Harrison & Oakland, 2003) • Ages & Stages Questionnaires, 3rd ed. (Squires & Bricker, 2009) • Ages & Stages Questionnaires–Social Emotional (Squires et al., 2002) • Assessment, Evaluation and Programming System for Infants and Children, 2nd ed. (Bricker & Waddell, 2002a) • Battelle Developmental Inventory, 2nd ed. (Newborg, 2004) • Bayley Scales of Infant and Toddler Development, 3rd ed. (Bayley, 2005) • Beery–Buktenica Developmental Test of Visual-Motor Integration, 6th ed. (Beery & Beery, 2010) • Behavior Assessment System for Children, 2nd ed. (Reynolds & Kamphaus, 2006) • Behavior Rating Inventory of Executive Function Preschool Version (Gioia et al., 2003) • Bruininks–Oseretsky Test of Motor Proficiency, 2nd ed. (Bruininks & Bruininks, 2005) • Carolina Curriculum for Infants and Toddlers with Special Needs, 3rd ed. (Johnson-Martin et al., 2004a) • Carolina Curriculum for Preschoolers with Special Needs, 2nd ed. (Johnson-Martin et al., 2004b) • Creative Curriculum for Infants, Toddlers and Twos (Dodge et al., 2011); for Preschool (Dodge et al., 2010) • Developmental Assessment of Young Children (Voress & Maddox, 2013) • Developmental Observation Checklist System (Hresko et al., 1998) • Developmental Pre-Feeding Checklist (Morris & Klein, 2000)

(Continued)

Table 4. Selected Assessments of Occupational Performance for Early Childhood (Birth–5 Years) *(Cont.)*

Domain of Occupational Therapy	Sample Assessments Used by Occupational Therapists

	• Developmental Test of Visual Perception (Hammill et al., 1993)
	• Early Coping Inventory (Zeitlin et al., 1988)
	• Early Learning Accomplishment Profile (Glover et al., 2002)
	• Erhardt Developmental Prehension Assessment (Erhardt, 1994)
	• Erhardt Developmental Vision Assessment (Erhardt, 1990)
	• Every Move Counts: Sensory-Based Communication Techniques (Korsten et al., 1993)
	• Gross Motor Function Measure (Russell et al., 2002)
	• HELP 3–6 Assessment (Teaford et al., 2010)
	• High Scope Child Observation Record (COR) for Infants and Toddlers (High Scope, 2002)
	    High Scope Preschool Curriculum (Epstein & Hohmann, 2012)
	• Infant/Toddler Sensory Profile (Dunn, 2002)
	• Inside HELP for 0~3 (Parks, 1992–2006)
	• Learning Accomplishment Profile (Hardin & Peisner-Feinberg, 2004)
	• Miller Assessment for Preschoolers (Miller, 1988)
	• Miller Function and Participation Scales (Miller, 2006)
	• Modified Checklist for Autism in Toddlers (M–CHAT; Robins et al., 1999)
	• Motor-Free Visual Perception Test, 3rd ed. (Colarusso & Hammill, 2003)
	• Ounce Scale (Marsden et al., 2003)
	• Peabody Developmental Motor Scales, 2nd ed. (Folio & Fewell, 2000)
	• Sensory Integration and Praxis Tests (Ayres, 1989)
	• Sensory Processing Measure–Preschool Home Form (Ecker & Parham, 2010); School Form
	    (Miller Kuhaneck et al., 2010)
	• Sensory Profile (Dunn, 1999)
	• Sensory Profile School Companion (Dunn, 2006)
	• Social Responsiveness Scale (Constantino & Gruber, 2005)
	• Test of Gross Motor Development, 2nd ed. (Ulrich, 2000)
	• Test of Visual–Motor Skills, 3rd ed. (Martin, 2010)
	• Test of Visual–Perceptual Skills 3 (Martin, 2006)

Performance Patterns	
• Habits • Routines • Roles • Rituals	• Activity-Based Assessment (Bricker et al., 1998) • Asset-Based Context Matrix (Wilson et al., 2004) • Canadian Occupational Performance Measure (Law et al., 2005) • Children's Assessment of Participation and Environment and Preferences for Activities of Children (King et al., 2005) • Routines-Based Interview Report Form (McWilliam, 2010)
Context	
• Cultural • Physical • Social • Personal • Temporal • Virtual	• Asset-Based Context Matrix (Wilson et al., 2004) • Canadian Occupational Performance Measure (Law et al., 2005) • Children's Assessment of Participation and Environment and Preferences for Activities of Children (King et al., 2005) • Early Childhood Environmental Rating Scale–Revised (Harms et al., 2005) • Home Observation for Measurement of the Environment–Revised (Caldwell & Bradley, 2001)

sources using multiple methods increases the reliability and validity of the information. As the occupational therapist analyzes the data collected, he or she may formulate one or more hypotheses. These hypotheses are based on the occupational therapist's knowledge, skills, and experiences as well as frames of reference within the profession. "Frames of reference provide the 'what' and 'how' of intervention and the theoretical perspectives provide the 'why'" (Handley-Moore & Chandler, 2007, p. 68).

Considering multiple frames of reference before establishing a hypothesis is important, because it guides the evaluation and intervention process. "A single occupational challenge looks very different from the perspectives each of these frames provides" (Candler, Clark, & Swinth, 2008, p. 19). When a skill, such as "not eating apples," is analyzed using frames of reference common to occupational thera-pists, different perspectives guide the assessment and intervention process. For example, if an occupational therapist uses a sensory processing/integrative framework and assumes a child is refusing to eat certain foods, such as an apple, because of sensory aversions (e.g., texture, smell), intervention planning would focus on increasing the child's ability to accept a wider range of textures and smells. However, if an occupational therapist uses a motor planning framework, intervention might focus on learning new motor skills so that the child can bite and chew apples.

Evaluating these hypotheses is critical in ruling out possible hypotheses not supported by data collected during the assessment process. The hypothesis supported by the data is used to effectively develop an intervention plan. Examples of various hypotheses are listed in Table 5.

Table 5. Using Frames of Reference When Evaluating a Hypothesis

Frame of Reference	Rationale	Intervention Focus
Behavior	Does not want to eat apples	Teach child how to put applesauce or baked apple in his mouth and immediately reward with a preferred behavior.
Biomechanical	Poor chewing and swallowing due to low tone in head/neck	Provide support for neck/chin alignment so he can chew/swallow a baked apple.
Cognitive	Does not understand if apples can be swallowed safely	Teach him how apples feel different when cooked or raw and how it feels in your mouth when you chew it.
Coping	Screams because he doesn't know how to respond	Teach him how to select a fruit he prefers.
Developmental	Hasn't developed necessary skills (e.g., rotary chewing)	Place food on molars to facilitate chewing.
Motor learning	Hasn't learned the skill	Daily practice alternating kinds of apples (e.g., sweet, crisp, baked) and occasionally provide him feedback.
Neurodevelopmental	Lacks ability to bring hand to mouth due to decreased postural tone	Use key points of control and guide hand movements.
Occupational	Environment does not support participation in lunch behaviors due to noise	Turn television off and encourage family to eat meals together at the table.
Sensory integration/processing	Finds texture or smell aversive	Work on increasing range of textures and smells.

The analysis of the child's occupational performance requires the occupational therapist understand the "complex and dynamic interaction among performance skills, performance patterns, contexts and environments, activity demands and client factors" (AOTA, 2008, p. 651). Within an evaluation, the occupational therapist identifies the supports and needs within areas of occupation; the demands of the activity within the client's context/environment; the client's values, beliefs, spirituality, body functions, and body structures that affect performance; and the client's actual performance skills and patterns. The influence of each of these aspects on early childhood areas of occupation will be discussed next.

Participation in Areas of Occupation

Young children with disabilities, or who are at risk for disabilities, may have limitations in performance in one or more area of occupation. Occupational therapists working with children in early childhood often focus on activities of daily living (ADLs), rest, play, social participation, and education. They also should consider the parent–child relationship during the evaluation and as part of the intervention plan (Humphry, 1989).

Current infant mental health practices focus on the dynamic relationship between parents/caregiver and a child under age 3 years (Schultz-Krohn & Cara, 2000). Interactions between the parent and child, as well as how the parent perceives the child, are important to understanding this relationship. "We must be astute observers and willing to see people in their milieu as we put on different lenses" (Swick & Williams, 2006, p. 375), including cultural, social, and economic factors that are part of their lives/systems. When working with young children, both the child and the family are clients, and the child–family relationship should be enhanced. Under IDEA, Part C (Infant & Toddler Program) requires a "family-directed assessment of the resources, priorities, and concerns of the family and the identification of supports and services necessary to enhance the family's capacity to meet the developmental needs of their infant or toddler" (§1436[a][2]).

Outcomes may be specific to the child or the family (e.g., the family needs a way to get the child to doctor's visits). Evaluation should include the child's participation in occupations as well as interactions with the family/caregivers that support or inhibit these occupations. Examples of common early childhood activities used to assess the specific areas of occupation can be found in Table 6.

ADLs

Self-care performance is a critical aspect of health and well-being of a child. Basic self-care skills develop during early childhood years and "are among the first achievements of childhood, and . . . provide independence, social approval and a sense of mastery for the child" (Henderson, 2006, p. 193). Self-care skills are dependent on motor development (e.g., postural control, oral–motor control, hand skills; Case-Smith, 2000b; Shepherd, 2001).

Occupational therapists use observation, as well as formal assessment methods, in natural or simulated environments to identify the child's strengths and needs in their ADLs. Examples of selected assessments for ADLs are included in Table 4. Observations; interviews with family, caregivers, and relevant others; and formal tools provide specific information about the child's typical performance and expectations within the setting.

Rest and Sleep

Krakowiak and colleagues (Krakowiak, Goodlin-Jones, Hertz-Picciotto, Croen, & Hansen, 2008) found that whereas 25% of typically developing children experience sleep problems, 53% of children with a diagnosis of ASD between the ages of 2 and 5 years had some type of sleep problem. Children with an ASD may have difficulty falling asleep or staying asleep as compared to peers (Allik, Larsson, & Smedje, 2006; Honomichl, Goodlin-Jones, Burnham, Gaylor, & Anders, 2002).

Table 6. Using the *Framework* (American Occupational Therapy Association, 2008) as a Guide for Evaluating Occupations

Area of Occupation	Examples of Early Childhood Activities (these refer to the child's performance and to building the capacity of the family/caregiver to meet their child's special needs)
Activities of daily living	Washing hands, dressing, eating, feeding, getting into sitting position, cleaning glasses, blowing nose, using toilet; family/caregiver can implement strategies to change diapers of child with high postural tone
Instrumental activities of daily living	Care of pet, using computers, putting toys away, riding in the car seat, riding in the seat in the grocery cart; family/caregiver can position child safely in grocery cart
Rest and sleep	Ability to relax during rest time, sleeping through the night, return to sleep by self if awaken, ability to self-soothe; family/caregiver will have several options to calm fussy child
Education	Preliteracy (looking at books, making strokes with crayon); early intervention: adaptive, cognitive, communication, physical, social, or emotional development; school: academic and developmental activities
Work	Functional work tasks (e.g., sorting, matching, stacking)
Play	Using a variety of toys and equipment, play exploration and participation (e.g., participating in games with rules)
Leisure	Free time use, dancing to music
Social participation	Interactions with family, peers, educational staff, and others

Note. Modified from "Evaluation, Assessment, and Outcomes in Early Childhood," by G. F. Clark, 2010, in *Early Childhood: Occupational Therapy Services for Children Birth to Five* (p. 151), B. Chandler (Ed.), Bethesda, MD: AOTA Press. Copyright © 2011 by the American Occupational Therapy Association. Adapted with permission.

These problems may include difficulty falling asleep, waking up during the night, and/or difficulty waking up in the morning.

If sleep patterns are disrupted for more than a week, this is considered a sleep problem (Durand, 1998). Documented reasons for sleep problems include seizures, gastrointestinal problems (e.g., reflux), and medication use (LaVesser & Hilton, 2010). Children with medical conditions may require tube feeding or suctioning during the evening or have problems (e.g., reflux, emotional, regulatory) that interfere with sleep (Shepherd, 2012). Disrupted sleep may cause family members to become sleep deprived and increase the risk of child abuse (Kodak & Piazza, 2008). Interviewing families about bedtime routines, strategies they use when the child wakes up, and environmental factors may provide insight that could help with intervention planning. Tools such as Sensory Profile (Dunn, 1999) and the Infant/Toddler Sensory Profile (Dunn, 2002) help provide some information about the influence of the child's sensory modulation and sensory processing on sleep.

Play

Play is a child's main occupation and thus should receive special attention during evaluation. Play influences the development of motor, social communication, cognitive, and self-care skills. Observing social interactions with people (e.g., turn-taking, sharing), cognitive skills (e.g., problem solving, imitation, attention, concentration) and motor skills (e.g., manipulating and releasing objects, jumping) provides insight into a child's abilities.

Assessment of play occurs through standardized and nonstandardized methods and typically includes structured observations. The Knox Preschool Play Scale (Knox, 2008) may be used when the occupational therapist wants to identify the types of play a child demonstrates. The Test of Playfulness (Skard & Bundy, 2008) may be used to examine a child's playfulness and motivation in unstructured play situations. Regardless of the method used, the therapist should identify *how* the child plays and *what* motivates him or her (e.g., interests, preferences).

Social Participation

Social participation emphasizes the child's and family members' ability to engage with each other. As the child's social circle broadens, the focus changes to include neighborhood and community relationships, especially peer relationships. Information about a child's social interactions with peers/friends, family, and at the community level (e.g., school, day care, library) is typically gathered through observation and interview. What opportunities does the child have to interact with peers or people outside of the family? How does the child initiate a conversation with another person? How does the child keep that conversation going, or does he or she end it? Does the child prefer interacting with an adult or a peer? To what degree are the child's cognitive, motor, language, and sensory processing skills supporting or impeding interactions?

Education

All states and U.S. territories currently participate in IDEA Part C, a federal grant program that provides early intervention to children under 3 years of age and their families. Children under 3 years of age with disabilities may receive special instruction services provided by early childhood teachers or, if children are eligible for Early Head Start, they may receive services from staff to promote early learning. IDEA requires that a formal transition plan be developed to help the child transition from Part C to preschool or appropriate services (§303.209 [a][1]) by his or her third birthday (except states that extend their Part C services to age 5 years).

Early childhood special education programs for 3- to 5-year-old children with disabilities (and peers, in inclusive preschool programs) provide academic and developmental activities. Child care centers and community preschools also may provide specific instruction in academics and preliteracy skills. In

recent years, responding to the need to improve math and science education in the United States, the push for science, technology, engineering, and mathematics education has been incorporated in early childhood programs (Katz, 2010).

Analysis of performance in preschool will depend on the school type, curriculum, instruction received, and the environment. Head Start, early childhood special education preschool programs, and private preschools all provide educational learning opportunities for young children but, because of agency or federal requirements, the emphasis of their program, training of their teachers, and expectations of the children may vary (e.g., Head Start has a parent support and training component, private preschools may be taught by educators with a 2-year degree, early childhood special education programs must follow IDEA and state law).

IDEA Part B evaluations require a statement of the child's present levels of academic achievement and functional performance, including how the child's disability affects his or her involvement and progress in the general education curriculum and how the disability affects his or her participation in appropriate activities (§1441[d][1][A][I]). Occupational therapists should understand the school routines, curricula being used in the setting, how instruction is being provided, and aspects of the educational environment that support or interfere with functioning across the school routines, including classroom, playground, bathrooms, lunch area, and so on. Being aware of the standards and expectations used within these settings (e.g., preschool rules and procedures, state or national standards) is important.

For occupational therapists working in preschool settings, observation of child performance during natural routines with peers, review of products (e.g., portfolio, work samples), and teacher interviews may not provide adequate information to determine discrepancy or programming needs. Additional information may be obtained by reviewing data gathered by the teacher (including curriculum-based assessments) or administration of formal measures (see Table 4).

Contexts and Environments

Occupational therapists acknowledge the influence of cultural, personal, temporal, virtual, physical, and social contextual factors on occupations and activities. *Contexts* are identified as cultural, personal, temporal, and virtual factors that exist within and around the person. *Environments* are those external physical and social factors that surround the person (AOTA, 2008).

Observations of the child's performance in and across multiple environments allow the occupational therapist to identify the contextual and environmental factors that support or hinder occupational performance. These observations of child performance during natural routines and contexts are used to structure the environment during interventions. Occupational therapy practitioners observe the child's performance in the current environment and consider challenges for the child in future environments as the child transitions to day care, preschool, kindergarten, or other locations.

Activity Demands

Determining whether a child is able to complete an activity depends not only on the performance skills, performance patterns, and client factors of an individual but also on the demands the activity itself places on the person. The *demands* of an activity are aspects of the activity that include the tools needed to carry out the activity, the space and social demands required by the activity, and the required actions and performance skills needed to take part in the given activity (AOTA, 2008).

As the child performs the activity, the occupational therapist analyzes the various demands of the activity, including the supports or modifications needed to increase successful performance. Grading and varying the demands of the activity and environment to provide a "just-right challenge" for the child, without exceeding his or her current level of skills, requires careful analysis of the activity and materials by the therapist during the evaluation and, later, dur-

ing intervention. When children with motor impairments need adaptive equipment or environmental modifications to participate in desired activities (e.g., modified spoons for self-feeding), the occupational therapist analyzes the need for adaptive equipment or assistive technology and balances the selected equipment and environmental modifications to the child's cognitive abilities.

Client Factors

Client factors are the underlying abilities, values, beliefs, and spirituality; body functions; and body structures that affect the individual's occupational performance (AOTA, 2008). The occupational therapist evaluates neuromusculoskeletal and movement-related functions, such as joint range of motion, reflexes, muscle tone, and postural alignment, to identify existing problems and implement intervention. Occupational therapy practitioners, with their holistic approach to clients, consider the influence of the children's and family's values, beliefs, and spirituality. These client factors (e.g., values or interests and beliefs, including fears) can hold the key to engagement in the therapy process and improved performance in desired activities and occupations. For example, if certain foods have caused intense stomachaches (e.g., gastrointestinal issues) in the past, a child may be afraid of eating because he or she believes that food causes his or her stomach to hurt. The family's values, beliefs, and spirituality may affect the child's development and performance (e.g., if a family believes bottle drinking is necessary for their 4-year-old son with CP to obtain fluids, they may not choose to work on cup drinking as a goal).

Performance Skills

The evaluation of children ages birth through 5 years includes overt and subtle factors that may affect performance. *Performance skills* are the observable, goal-directed actions by which an individual engages in occupation. These can be subdivided into motor and praxis, sensory–perceptual, cognitive processing, emotional regulatory, and communication and social skills (AOTA, 2008). Depending on the medical diagnosis or disability, one or more of these performance skills could be affected. Unlike the body functions that reflect capacities that reside inside the body, performance skills are abilities demonstrated by the child (AOTA, 2008). For example, emotional regulation skills can be observed through the child's behaviors during sleep/rest or when expressing emotions. Many assessments for young children focus on developmental milestones; however, the occupational therapist also must make observations regarding the qualitative aspects of motor control and performance.

A child may be able to use scissors to cut across a paper (milestone); however, the child had to stand to complete the task, held the scissors incorrectly, had excessive saliva loss that dampened the entire front of his or her shirt, and snipped a finger holding the paper. Even though the child completed the task of cutting across the paper, the quality begs further exploration. Examples of performance skills in early childhood are presented on Table 7.

Motor and Praxis Skills

Assessment of motor (including gross motor, fine motor, and oral–motor skills, as well as ideation, initiation, and the planning and execution of novel actions) may be completed during play-based

Table 7. Examples of Performance Skills and Performance Patterns (American Occupational Therapy Association, 2008)

Area	Early Intervention Examples	Preschool Examples
Performance Skills		
Emotional regulation	• Difficulty with sleeping, feeding, self-calming • Displays appropriate emotions, such as laughing or smiling	• High arousal and unusual sensory-seeking behaviors (e.g., can't attend for more than 5 s; always on the move) • Responding to other people's feeling
Motor and praxis	• Manipulating spoon to bring food to mouth • Squatting down to retrieve a toy	• Coordinating body to climb on playground equipment • Drawing shapes
Sensory–perceptual	• Locating parent's voice in a crowd • Discerning hot and cold food temperatures	• Identifying rough and smooth objects • Selecting correct piece to fit into puzzle
Cognitive	• Anticipating events that occur frequently • Identifying familiar toys	• Sequencing tasks to complete three-step commands
Communication and social	• Imitating other people's actions • Gesturing to make needs known	• Taking turns during play with others • Fulfilling the role as "line leader"
Performance Patterns		
Habits (automatic)	• Using pacifier for calming • Dumping all toys out of toy box before playing	• Sleeping with stuffed toy • Spitting out foods that has chunks
Routines	• Getting ready for bed routines • Feeding schedule	• Circle time, play centers, lunch time, rest time
Rituals (symbolic)	• Putting on mother's shoes to walk around house	• Kissing parent when saying goodbye
Roles	• Child • Family member	• Student, peer

Note. Modified from "Evaluation, Assessment, and Outcomes in Early Childhood," by G. F. Clark, 2010, in *Early Childhood: Occupational Therapy Services for Children Birth to Five* (p. 151–152), B. Chandler (Ed.), Bethesda, MD: AOTA Press. Copyright © 2011 by the American Occupational Therapy Association. Adapted with permission.

assessments, curriculum-based measures, parent report, and standardized tools (see Table 4). Postural stability, mobility, gross motor skills, strength, coordination, motor planning, neurodevelopment, and neuromuscular status are frequently included in *gross motor* assessments. *Fine motor* assessments include prehension patterns, isolation of finger movements, dexterity, manipulation, bilateral hand use, and tool use (Mulligan, 2003). Structured observations of fine motor performance are included in Table 8. Observations should include the quality of motor coordination and praxis skills. Motor planning praxis skills typically are evaluated through imitation such as gestures and postures (May-Benson, 2010) and as a child engages in novel or challenging tasks.

During the early years, important *oral–motor skills* develop. Eating or feeding is a critical occupation and skill and should be screened in all young children. Box 2 provides some questions that could be used during family interviews to identify strengths and barriers in eating and drinking performance. Evaluation may include observing the child's ability to swallow (e.g., coordinate suck/swallow/breathe, swallow to clear airway, swallow consecutively when drinking); drink (e.g., bottle, cup, straw); eat (e.g., suck, lateralize food, bite, chew); actions of tongue, lips, and cheeks during eating; range of foods in diet; and graphing of the young child's height and weight on a growth chart (CDC, 2012b).

Sensory–Perceptual Skills

The *Framework* (AOTA, 2008) defines *sensory–perceptual skills* as "actions or behaviors a client uses to locate, identify, and respond to sensations and to select, interpret, associate, organize, and remember sensory events via sensations" (p. 640). Sensory

Table 8. Structured Observations of Fine Motor Performance

Foundation Area	Example Observations

Hand Dominance	• Does the child demonstrate use of a dominant hand, mixed dominance, or ambiguous dominance?
	• If the child has mixed or no dominance:
	  • Does he or she avoid crossing midline?
	  • Does he or she consistently accomplish certain tasks (e.g., self-feeding, color) with one hand?

Grasp and Prehension Patterns	• Does the child have adequate hand strength to hold onto objects? • Does the child have difficulty grading pressure (too much or too little) when holding objects? • Can the child isolate finger motions to pick up smaller objects? • Does the quality of the child's grasp and prehension abilities differ when he or she is grasping or manipulating an object vs. using the object in a functional task?
Manipulation Skill	• What is the quality of the child's in-hand manipulation skill? • Can the child transition objects in his or her hand utilizing transverse palmar (palm-to-finger and finger-to-palm) motions, or does he or she stabilize the object against the table or him- or herself and regrasp? • Does the child demonstrate different manipulation abilities when he or she is grasping, carrying, or manipulating an object vs. using the object in a functional task?
Purposes and Quality of a Child's Interactions With Objects	• Does the child manipulate objects primarily for sensory gratification or for purposeful toy play? • Are tremors present, or do the child's movements appear ataxic? • Does the child have a hard time damping his or her reach? • Does the child frequently shift his or her position while interacting with an object, or does he or she frequently turn or reposition a task? • If so, is he or she doing so to avoid midline crossing or for visual inspection? • Does the child use peripheral vision or central vision, or does he or she accomplish tasks "by feel"?

Note. From "Occupational Therapy Process for Individuals With an ASD," in *Occupational Therapy Practice Guidelines for Children and Adolescents With Autism* (p. 25), S. Tomcheck & J. Case-Smith, Bethesda, MD: AOTA Press. Copyright © 2009 by the American Occupational Therapy Association. Used with permission.

Box 2. Sample Interview Questions to Understand Feeding and Eating Skills

1. Who usually feeds this child? (List all primary feeders.)
2. What is the child's primary method of food intake (e.g., oral, tube)?
3. What equipment or utensils does the child use for eating or drinking?
4. Describe the child's typical meal and amount of food eaten and liquid drank.
5. What times during the day does the child eat?
6. How long does it take for the child to eat in one meal?
7. Does the child typically eat meats, vegetables, fruits, dairy, and carbohydrates?
8. What are foods or liquids typically eaten at (home, day care, school) that you would like this child to eat?
9. What do you feel are strengths in this child's eating and drinking?
10. What do you feel are challenges in this child's eating and drinking?
11. What are your goals for this child (i.e., what would you like this child to be able to do)?

---

perception includes auditory, gustatory, olfactory, proprioceptive, tactile, vestibular, and visual sensations. When deficiencies are present in one or more systems, occupational performance is affected. Evaluators must understand the relationship between the child's performance and sensations during the activity or within the environment.

Both standardized measures and informal methods (e.g., observation, interviews, checklists) can be used to gather information about sensory perceptions within daily life situations. The Sensory Profile tests (Dunn, 1999, 2002) and Sensory Processing Measures (Ecker & Parham, 2010; Parham & Ecker, 2007) are standardized questionnaires that examine the child's sensory processing. Scores on the Sensory Profile reveal the child's typical sensory-processing patterns and their possible impact on daily occupational performance. The Sensory Processing Measures (home and preschool) provide information about the child's performance in various settings in their environment. Structured observations of the child's sensory–perceptual skills provide additional information and can be used to support formal or informal tools. Blanche (2002) developed structural observations of sensory-processing and praxis skills that can be used to evaluate children's ability to successfully participate in their daily occupations and activities.

Emotional Regulation

Emotional regulation is described as "actions or behaviors a client uses to identify, manage, and express feelings while engaged in activities or interacting with others" (AOTA, 2008, p. 640). Evaluation of this complex process requires measurement of the child's behavior patterns and skills and sensory processing. Observations of behaviors such as emotional reactivity to stimuli, ability to calm or recover following intense response, and the match between an emotional response and contextual factors are important aspects of emotion regulation assessment. Assessments may be used to measure the child's sensory processing at school or home as well as the individual's coping skills (see Table 4).

Cognitive Skills

Children's cognitive skills include behaviors or actions they use to plan and manage their performance during activities (AOTA, 2008). Early cognitive development includes attention (and joint attention), memory, object permanence, causality, imitation, problem solving, and sorting objects. Occupational therapists understand the influence of cognitive abilities on performance. Many curriculum-based measures include cognitive development, but an observation of these abilities during the child's functional performance is also important. Assessment tools for this area are listed in Table 4.

Communication and Social Skills

Children use various actions or behaviors to communicate and interact with others in their environment (AOTA, 2008; Fisher, 2006). The ability to communicate with others is critical for social relationships and participation.

The assessment of young children's communication skills is typically performed by a speech–language pathologist or an early childhood educator; however, occupational therapists understand communication difficulties and their impact on the child's performance. Children with communication delays may exhibit behaviors such as withdrawal, low self-confidence, frustration, or anxiety. Working collaboratively with speech–language pathologists, occupational therapy practitioners can reinforce therapy goals to enhance the child's communication and social interactions.

Serious challenging social behaviors in young children have increased significantly over the past 10 years (Knitzer, 2002; Shonkoff & Phillips, 2000). Dunlap, Lewis, and McCart (2006) found early childhood behaviors are associated with poor social skills, academic performance, and social adjustment (S. B. Campbell, 1995). Identifying problems in social skills early, before patterns of resistance and aggression develop, is critical. For young children, the primary relationships exist between the child and caregiver. Evaluations during this age group focus on attachment to family or objects, expressions of emotion, and participation in simple games (e.g., peek-a-boo). During ages 2 through 4 years, children typically become more independent as they move around their environment. Relationships with siblings, peers, and other adults become important. Peer play and environmental exploration emerge as children seek new experiences. As children develop trust in the environment and language skills, their autonomous nature is strengthened (Case-Smith, 2010).

Screening tools such as Ages & Stages Questionnaires–Social Emotional (Squires,

Bricker, & Twombly, 2002) can be used in home, school, medical, or community locations. Assessment of social skills can be conducted formally and through structured observations (see Table 4). The natural observation of the child during play can yield information about the child's interactions with peers, siblings, and adults. Understanding the expectations, rules, and management of conflict in each of the child's settings provides the occupational therapist with knowledge that can be used for intervention planning. IDEA requires the evaluation of social–emotional skills for every child who is referred for eligibility under Part C.

Performance Patterns

Performance patterns are "behaviors related to daily life activities that are habitual or routine" (AOTA, 2008); they include habits, routines, rituals, and roles (see Table 7). "Naturally occurring family routines and meaningful rituals provide both a predictive structure that guides behavior and an emotional climate that supports early development" (Spagnola & Fiese, 2007, p. 284). When evaluating habits, routines, and rituals in a very young child, the occupational therapist must understand that the family or caregiver often sets these routines (e.g., bedtime, eating, bathing, going to the store), but during the preschool years, the children begin establishing some routines as well ("I will do it"). Occupational therapists should determine whether these routines, habits, and rituals promote or hinder the child's participation and health. For example, a child who requires medications or medical treatments on a specific schedule may be unable to participate in preschool events during these procedures or could become ill if the routine is altered.

Case studies illustrating occupational therapy evaluation and intervention process with children age 0 through 5 years are presented in Table 9. The complexity of the family and child's needs demonstrate the need for services from skilled occupational therapists and occupational therapy assistants.

Table 9. Application of the Guidelines: Examples of Evaluation and Intervention for Children With Feeding/Eating, Social–Emotional, and Motor Delays

Description of Client	Occupational Therapy Evaluation	Occupational Therapy Intervention
• **Juan** is 11 months old and was referred to early intervention program by his gastroenterologist due to severe refusal to eat foods orally. • Evaluation by early intervention team indicates some delays in Juan's adaptive skills, but cognitive, communication, physical, and social–emotional skills were on target for his adjusted age. • Feeding was the primary concern. Parents stated Juan's pediatrician told them to put foods into his mouth and he would swallow them eventually. Instead they found Juan spit the food out and screamed when they came near him with food. • Parents state Juan is a curious and easy baby, except for mealtime.	• Interview with Juan's mother indicated Juan was born at 28 weeks and had surgery for a fundoplication and gastrostomy tube due to retching (acid reflux) and poor sucking skills. Parent reports Juan screams if she tries to feed him by mouth. Tube feedings are his primary source of nutrition. • Structured observation of Juan during snack was conducted to identify aspects of the environment, activity demands, performance skills, and performance patterns that were supporting or preventing feeding skills. • The Developmental Pre-Feeding Checklist (Morris & Klein, 2000) was used to specifically identify oral–motor strengths and needs. • Evaluation results indicated Juan would touch some food items but screamed if they were brought near his face. He will allow a pacifier, toothbrush, and his/adult's fingers in his mouth. Delayed tongue mobility, lip closure, chewing/biting, delayed swallow were observed. • Family goals: Juan will eat food and drink liquids.	• Juan's pediatrician and gastroenterologist have approved the occupational therapy's feeding plan for Juan and receive updates regarding Juan's performance. • The occupational therapist, family, and nutritionist have phone conversations once a month to discuss his progress. • Occupational therapy services are provided weekly in the home prior to Juan's noon tube feeding so that he was hungry. • Coaching model of service delivery allows family and occupational therapist to work as partners to problem-solve solutions and strategies for Juan (Fraser et al., 2004; Haywood & McCann, 2009). • Family and occupational therapist agree to initiate sensory exploration of food, develop oral–motor skills, and use behavioral reinforcements while allowing Juan to initiate oral play with food (Gaebler & Hanzlik, 1996; Jadcherla et al., 2009; White-Traut et al., 2002). • Tube feedings continue as scheduled.
• **Wendy** is an almost-4-year-old child who attends the preschool program for children with special needs. • She was recently referred because she continues to drink from a bottle and will run if nonpreferred foods are placed near her on the table. • Wendy has a diagnosis of developmental delay and is functioning at about 18-month level of development.	• Interview with the family indicates that eating has always been a struggle. They feed Wendy the same foods on the same plate every day to decrease resistance. A special formula has been prescribed for her for weight gain. Parents are concerned about her developmental delays. • Reviewed the teacher's data regarding Wendy's current curricular assessment of developmental skills. • Interviewed the parent and teacher regarding Wendy's participation in home/preschool meals. • Observed Wendy, her peers, and educational staff during snack in the preschool.	• Occupational therapist will provide services 60 min/month. Services will include working with Wendy to on skill building, attending team meetings to problem-solve with educational staff and parents, training school personnel in strategies that can be integrated into Wendy's daily routine (Dunst et al., 2006). • Strategies incorporate aspects of behavior (reinforcement) to increase range of food eaten (Benoit et al., 2000; Greer et al., 2008; Williams et al., 2007). • Wendy is immediately reinforced with highly preferred food when she touches or tastes nonpreferred foods.

(Continued)

Table 9. Application of the Guidelines: Examples of Evaluation and Intervention for Children With Feeding/Eating, Social–Emotional, and Motor Delays *(Cont.)*

Description of Client	Occupational Therapy Evaluation	Occupational Therapy Intervention
	• Data gathered indicate Wendy will independently put her bottle and crisp, crunchy foods (e.g., dry cereal, chips) into her mouth. She will not allow any cups/straws near her mouth and will leave the table when smelly (e.g., bananas) foods or blended foods (e.g., applesauce, pudding) are near her. She refuses to put her fingers in anything that is "slippery/slimy." • Family and school goal: Wendy will eat snacks offered at school and drink from a cup.	• Strategies include shaping cup-drinking behaviors to increase skills in this area (Laud et al., 2009; Wilder et al., 2005). • Education and training are provided to parents, teacher, and paraprofessional by occupational therapist.
• **Tyrone** is a 2-year-old boy who received early intervention, including occupational therapy services, in another state before moving to his current state. • He was born at 28 weeks' gestation and diagnosed with cerebral palsy. Tyrone primarily uses his right arm for batting at objects and sits if supported. Head control is delayed. He will interact by smiling or crying but has no other verbal sounds. • Family is requesting an occupational therapy evaluation from a community-based clinic as well as through an early intervention team. • Tyrone's mother works part-time, so he is at a child care center on Tuesdays and Thursdays.	Occupational therapist on early intervention team: • As part of the early intervention team, all areas of Tyrone's development in the home were evaluated using family interview, observation, and curriculum-based measures. • Participated in the family assessment using Routines-Based Interview Report Form (McWilliam, 2010) to identify family routines, activities, concerns, and priorities. • Conducted interview with day care provider and structured observation during free playtime and table activities. Obtained preschool schedule of activities. Occupational therapist in community-based clinic: • Used data from early intervention evaluation report to identify specific areas for further assessment. • Reviewed routines, activities, concerns, and priorities gathered from early intervention team with family for intervention planning in clinic. • With a speech-language pathologist, specifically evaluated skills in communication, physical, and self-help through parent interview, structured observations, and a standardized assessment. Summary • Evaluation results reveal significant delays in all areas of development (e.g., physical, cognitive, adaptive, communication, social–emotional) that interfered with his ability to participate in family and child care center's activities, including play, moving independently, and social interactions.	• The occupational therapists and family agreed to coordinate therapy across environments and to prepare Tyrone for transitioning to his next setting, preschool (Dankert et al., 2003). • Early intervention occupational therapy services are provided 45 min/week in the home or child care (alternating settings); medical-based occupational therapy services at the community-based clinic are provided 45 min/week (Bierman et al., 2008; Bruder, 1997; Love et al., 2005). • Strategies include interventions focused on improving motor and cognitive skills in order to participate in play and pre-academic skills at the child care center (e.g., looking at books, building with various materials, using various technology). • Parent and teacher education was provided in all settings with written documentation that could be shared among providers. • The occupational therapy assistant employed by the early intervention agency provided services during the natural routines (e.g., opening group, playground, building centers, art, play at home) to enhance Tyrone's participation during family and day care activities (Bruder, 2003; Dunst et al., 2006). Intervention was based on the activities chosen by the children. • The occupational therapist employed at a community clinic used play among parent, child, and therapist to enhance Tyrone's participation and engagement in various activities (Law et al., 2011).

(Continued)

Table 9. Application of the Guidelines: Examples of Evaluation and Intervention for Children With Feeding/Eating, Social–Emotional, and Motor Delays *(Cont.)*

Description of Client	Occupational Therapy Evaluation	Occupational Therapy Intervention
	• Family goals: Tyrone will continue to grow and develop new skills so he can play and use his hands when he gets to preschool.	• Early literacy was emphasized during intervention by using materials common in his home, day care, and upcoming preschool environments (e.g., books, alphabet letters, shapes, games, computers and electronic devices, prewriting and writing tasks) to build skills needed for reading and writing.
• **Larkin** is a 2-year-old boy attending an Early Head Start center-based program. • He frequently behaves aggressively toward his peers, hitting if he does not get his way and pushing children out of his way. • Larkin enjoys rough-and-tumble play but often accidently hurts his playmates.	• Evaluation of sensory processing using the Infant/Toddler Sensory Profile (Dunn, 2002). • Evaluation of motor development conducted using standardized assessment. • Interviewed caregiver, teacher/staff to determine typical antecedents and consequences of this behavior. • Observations of social interactions and play skills during structured and less structured playtimes. Summary • Evaluation results revealed deficits in sensory modulation on the Sensory Profile that are affecting Larkin's ability to interact with his peers during less-structured play times.	• Weekly occupational therapy groups using peer modeling, reinforcement, and direct instruction to enhance social participation (Vaughn et al., 2003). • Social stories explaining the perspective of child's peers and appropriate physical play (Crozier & Tincani, 2007). • Conference with parent, teacher, and staff to explain Larkin's sensory-processing strengths and needs, make modifications to environment, and discuss strategies to enhance Larkin's sensory-processing skills (Bierman et al., 2008; Dankert et al., 2003). • Model and reinforce appropriate coping strategies for 2-year-old. • Discuss the use of massage before bed and nap times with the family (Escalona et al., 2001; von Knorring et al., 2008).
• **Lilli** is a 5-year-old girl attending kindergarten at her local public school. • She plays alone at recess, frequently complaining that no one likes her. In the classroom, she does not follow rules and frequently cuts in front of the line. During free time, Lilli does not engage in play with the other kids; instead, she sits in the corner with a stuffed animal. • Lilli has difficulty visually referencing her peers and interacting with peers beyond one verbal exchange.	• Evaluate play skills using the Knox Pre-School Play Scale (Knox, 2008). • Evaluate performance in motor, visual–motor, and social–emotional areas using the M-Fun, teacher interview, parent interview, and observations. • Structured observations during recess and free play times in the classroom. Summary: • Lilli demonstrates significant delays in her ability to approach peers to initiate play and the skills to sustain play beyond one exchange.	• Bimonthly occupational therapy intervention in the school setting training teacher/staff to use various strategies during Lilli's school routines (Bierman et al., 2008; Dunst et al, 2006). 　• Using principles of positive behavior intervention strategies, review with Lilli the classroom rules, and praise her when she follows them. 　• Use strategies including social stories, modeling, and contingent reinforcement (Crozier & Tincani, 2007; Vaughn et al., 2003). • Design visual schedules for less-structured playtimes (Betz et al., 2008). • Provide practice situations for kids to engage with Lilli in structured play areas with an adult to guide the interactions (Kim et al., 2003; Tanta et al., 2005). • Discuss with parents the option of community social training groups.

Occupational Therapy Intervention and Evidence-Based Practice in Early Childhood

Occupational therapy practitioners use the information gathered collaboratively with the client during the evaluation process (e.g., occupational profile and analysis of occupational performance) to facilitate engagement in occupation related to participation and health through interventions that are client-centered and occupation-based (AOTA, 2008) and, in the case of early intervention, family-centered. Eligibility and interventions vary according to the client and the context of service delivery (Moyers & Dale, 2007). A family's insurance company may provide reimbursement for occupational therapy interventions for a specific number of visits and then deny further funding for intervention. Under IDEA (2004), children must be eligible for state early intervention services (Part C) or special education (Part B) before occupational therapy intervention can be provided. To maximize client engagement and participation, interventions should be focused on outcomes desired by the client (e.g., child, family, caregiver, teacher) and be based on current evidence.

Intervention

Throughout the intervention process, information from the evaluation is integrated with evidence from the literature, professional judgment, client values, theory, frame of reference, and practice. There are three steps to the intervention process: (1) the intervention plan, (2) intervention implementation, and (3) intervention review. Each of these will be discussed in further detail.

Intervention Plan

The intervention plan design is directed by six factors: (1) the client's goals, values, and beliefs; (2) the client's health and well-being; (3) the client's performance skills and performance patterns; (4) the collective influence of the context, environment, activity demands, and client factors on the client's performance; (5) the context in which the intervention is provided; and (6) the best available evidence to meet the identified outcomes (AOTA, 2008). The intervention plan documents the goals that were developed collaboratively with the client (e.g., family teacher, caregiver), the intervention approaches, and types of interventions (AOTA, 2008). The intervention plan also should include the expected frequency, duration, and intensity of the intervention; the location of the intervention; and the anticipated discharge environment (Moyers & Dale, 2007).

AOTA's (2010) *Standards of Practice for Occupational Therapy* state that the occupational therapist is responsible for the documentation of the intervention plan within the time frames, formats, and standards established by the practices settings and relevant laws and regulatory and payer requirements. Occupational therapists working in early intervention and school settings must complete professional intervention plans. Documents such as the IFSP or IEP outline family/child outcomes or student goals but do not meet the professional requirements of an occupational therapy intervention plan.

On the basis of the targeted goals, the occupational therapy practitioner determines the intervention approach that is best suited to address the client's goals (which may include IFSP outcomes and IEP goals). The intervention approaches include

- *Create or promote.* This approach provides enriched contextual activity experiences to enhance performance in natural contexts (Dunn, McClain, Brown, & Youngstrom, 1998), such as promoting social participation for a young child by facilitating family participation in community play groups at their library or church.
- *Establish and restore.* This intervention approach is designed to support the development of client variables to establish a skill or ability that has not yet developed or to restore a skill or ability that has been impaired (Dunn et al., 1998), such as facilitating the development of oral–motor skills so that a child is able to bite and chew foods during meals.
- *Maintain.* In this approach, performance and health that the young child has previously (re)gained are preserved (AOTA, 2008); for example, a toddler with a head injury will maintain attention and imitation skills to sort simple objects.
- *Modify.* This approach involves adjusting activity demands and the contexts in which activities are performed to support safe, independent performance of valued activities (AOTA, 2008), for example, modifying a spoon and cup so the child is able to eat and drink independently during snack.
- *Prevent.* This is an intervention approach designed to address clients with or without disability who are at risk for occupational performance problems (Dunn et al., 1998), for example, planning intervention to prevent

social isolation and increase safety by providing education to the family on strategies to minimize the child's severe emotional outbursts and support the child's positive behaviors.

Intervention Implementation

Implementing the plan is the skilled process of altering factors in the client, activity, context, and environment to effect positive change in the client's engagement in occupation, participation, and health (AOTA, 2008). Interventions may focus on a single or several aspects of the domain (e.g., specific performance skill, performance pattern, context). The dynamic interrelationship between the child's performance and intervention, ongoing assessment, and intervention planning continue throughout the implementation process.

Occupational therapy practitioners determine the types of interventions for the most effective treatment based on available evidence and implement these interventions during the intervention approach identified on the plan. The types of interventions include the following:

- *Therapeutic use of self:* an occupational therapy practitioner's planned use of his or her personality, insights, perceptions, and judgments as a part of the therapeutic process (adapted from Punwar & Peloquin, 2000, p. 285);
- *Therapeutic use of occupations and activities*, which includes three different levels of activities: (1) occupation-based activity (e.g., putting a coat on to go outside with one's family, getting into a bathtub to take a bath); (2) purposeful activity (e.g., practice writing name, practice manipulating clothing fasteners), and (3) preparatory methods (e.g., fine motor exercises, orthotics/splints, sensory enrichment);
- *Consultation*, whereby the occupational therapy practitioner shares knowledge and expertise with others; however, the practitioner is not directly responsible for the outcome (Dunn, 2000, p. 113);

- *Education:* the occupational therapy practitioner imparts knowledge and information but does not result in the actual performance of the occupation/activity (AOTA, 2008); and
- *Advocacy:* the promotion of occupational justice and client empowerment to seek and obtain resources to fully participate in their daily life occupations (AOTA, 2008).

Although not all types of occupational therapy interventions are used for all approaches, the therapeutic use of self (i.e., therapist's use of his or her personality, perception, and judgment; AOTA, 2008) is an overarching concept that should be considered in each therapeutic interaction. Therapeutic use of self is a vital responsibility of the occupational therapy practitioner as well as of all members of the health care team.

Ongoing assessment to monitor the client's progress toward goals is conducted during this time. Results of assessments should be used to make decisions about changes in interventions. "In education settings, occupational therapists use formative and summative evaluation methods to gather data for decision making" (Clark, 2010, p. 743). *Formative evaluation* identifies progress in instructional program and answers the question "Is the intervention working?" whereas *summative evaluation* data identify performance at a specific point in time (e.g., at the end of the year, at the IEP review) and answers the overall question "Did the plan work?" For example, Rose's occupational therapist and teacher collect data twice a week in the preschool classroom to determine whether the intervention is improving Rose's performance (formative evaluation). To prepare for Rose's annual IEP meeting, the occupational therapist and teacher summarize Rose's progress (summative evaluation) to make decisions about her performance, determine outcomes, and identify needs to be addressed by the occupational therapist (Clark, 2010).

Intervention Review

Intervention review is a continuous process of reevaluating and reviewing the intervention plan, the effectiveness of its delivery, progress toward targeted outcomes, and the need for future occupational therapy and referrals to other agencies or professionals (AOTA, 2008). This regular monitoring of the results of occupational therapy intervention determines the need to continue or modify the intervention plan, discontinue intervention, provide follow-up, or refer the clients to other agencies or professionals.

Reevaluation may involve readministering assessments used at the time of initial evaluation, parent or client interviews, or a questionnaire that evaluates the status of each client. Reevaluation normally substantiates progress toward goal attainment, indicates any change in functional status, and directs modification to the intervention plan, if necessary (Moyers & Dale, 2007). In addition, this review of intervention may require revisiting available literature if occupational performance of the individual has changed.

Intervention review for young children is an ongoing process and is greatly influenced by the setting and context. For example, under IDEA, occupational therapy practitioners working in Part C/early intervention programs conduct ongoing assessment as part of the intervention process and as members of the multi- or interdisciplinary team; under Part B, the IEP team reviews the IEP at least annually, establishing new goals and outlining changes specifically designed instruction to address these goals. When children receive private services from occupational therapy practitioners, intervention review and outcome monitoring may be influenced by external factors, such as payer requirements.

After the intervention review, the occupational therapist may decide to continue services (modification of the plan, if applicable), begin transition planning, discontinue services, or make a referral to other services. These decisions should be based on data about client performance and follow regulations and procedures within the work setting. Teams are often involved in this process. For example, the IEP team makes the final decision about related services (e.g., occupational therapy) that are necessary for the child to benefit from their educational program.

Transition

Transitions are "actions coordinated to prepare for or facilitate a change, such as from one functional level to another, from one life [change] to another, from one program to another, or from one environment to another" (AOTA, 1998, p. 866). Children transition throughout their early years to different environments or programs (e.g., home to day care, home to preschool, preschool to kindergarten) and situations (e.g., change in occupational therapists, new siblings, parent divorce, moving to new home). Children with ongoing medical conditions may frequently transition between services in their home and the hospital. Occupational therapists may transition their services from a child's home or hospital to more community-located environments as the child attends child care or preschool.

Some early childhood transitions are mandated by law. IDEA Part C requires that transitioning for children turning 3 begin "not fewer than 90 days before the third birthday of the toddler with a disability if that toddler may be eligible for preschool services under Part B of the Act" (§303.209[b][i]). Transition options from Part C may include Part B special education programming (early childhood preschool programs with or without related services) or community resources (e.g., community preschools, preschool library activities for social skills). Although transition planning from preschool to kindergarten is not mandated under educational law, families and children may perceive the move into a more academic program to be a big step.

During any transitions, occupational therapy practitioners support positive transitions to prepare the family and child for changes in roles and routines and facilitate performance skills needed in next environment and context. The occupational therapy practitioner may provide information to the family about the new program, explain how expectations for the child will change, and facilitate communication with the providers of the child's future programs, when applicable.

If the child has medical concerns or medications, the occupational therapist may work collaboratively with the school nurse so that a health care plan is in place before the child begins school. Families with children who have health care needs, such as allergies, asthma, or seizures, should be encouraged to meet with the school nurse and identify training that is necessary for the teaching staff. For example, the school nurse could provide training on seizures, such as how to identify a seizure and what to do if someone has a seizure. Ongoing communication with team members, including the family, is important to identifying ongoing needs and plan for a smooth transition.

Discharge Planning, Discontinuation, and Follow-Up

Like transition, discontinuing and discharging services requires planning and should begin at the time services are initiated. Occupational therapists may recommend discontinuation of occupational therapy services when the child has met his or her goals and no additional goals are appropriate, services are no longer are needed because development is not significantly discrepant from expectations, at the request of the family, or if the child is unable to participate because of medical or health difficulties (AOTA, 2008). If the child receives services under IDEA, the occupational therapist, as part of the IEP team, may recommend discontinuation of occupational therapy services. Bundy (1995) stated that if there is no "goal [outcome] explicitly related to therapeutic areas of expertise . . . and no acknowledged need for consultation or staff training, then there is no educationally relevant justification for an OT . . . to provide any service to that student" (p. 70). For children under 3 years of age who received occupational therapy services on their IFSP, occupational therapy may be discontinued when the child and family outcomes no longer require the expertise of an occupational therapist, the family feels they have the capacity to meet their child's needs, concerns with the child's health or development cease to be problematic, or therapy is contraindicated due to medical reasons.

Follow-up is important to consider during discharge planning. If, in the future, the child's participation in daily life skills is negatively affected by changes in development, health, or context/environments, families may consider a new request for occupational therapy to determine whether services should be reinitiated. In addition to a formal request, routine screenings may be conducted within various settings. In a preschool setting, ongoing educational screenings may identify need for occupational therapy evaluation. Private clinics and diagnostic centers may conduct well-baby screenings or high-risk nursery follow-up visits to monitor developmental progress and provide recommendations. In addition, some settings may conduct formal surveys via phone, letter, or questionnaire as part of ongoing quality assurance programs. In any case, follow-up is an important yet often forgotten component of the occupational therapy process.

Documentation, Billing, and Reimbursement

Occupational therapy practitioners document intervention and client progress toward goals "within the time frames, formats, and standards established by practice settings, agencies, external accreditation programs, and payers" (AOTA, 2010, p. S109). Occupational therapy documentation meets four purposes:

1. It articulates the rationale for the provision of services and their relationship to the client's outcomes.

2. It reflects the therapist's clinical reasoning and professional judgment.
3. It communicates information about the client from an occupational therapy perspective.
4. It creates a chronological record of client status, occupational therapy services provided, and client outcomes (AOTA, 2013).

The following types of documentation may be completed for each client, as required by law, the practice setting, third-party payers, or some combination of these:

- Evaluation or screening report
- Occupational therapy service contacts
- Occupational therapy intervention plan
- Progress report
- Prescriptive/recommendation for adaptive equipment
- Reevaluation report
- Discharge or discontinuation report (AOTA, 2013).

Readers should refer to the *Guidelines for Documentation of Occupational Therapy* (AOTA, 2013) for specific report contents and fundamental elements of documentation.

Occupational therapists need to document how the child's problems affect functional behaviors and engagement in daily occupations and write intervention plans with clear goals that are objective, functional, and measurable (Hinojosa & Foto, 2004). This documentation can aid in obtaining reimbursement for occupational therapy services provided in medical and educational settings (e.g., school districts may bill Medicaid for occupational therapy services). Guidelines for occupational therapy evaluation and intervention billing using *Current Procedural Terminology*^{TM} codes (American Medical Association, 2012) can be found in Appendix B.

Outcomes

Occupational therapy practitioners believe that active engagement in occupation is necessary to promote, facilitate, and maintain health and participation (AOTA, 2008; Moyers & Dale, 2007). Occupational therapy outcomes are "focused on how people live with health conditions and how the individual can achieve a productive, fulfilling life" (Baum & Christiansen, 2005, p. 527, as cited in Moyers & Dale, 2007). These outcomes reflect the end result of occupational therapy but should be interwoven throughout the process.

The *Framework* (AOTA, 2008) outlines two steps to implementing the outcome process. First, select the type of outcomes and measures, including, but not limited to, occupational performance, adaptation, health and wellness, participation, prevention, self-advocacy, quality of life, and occupational justice. Second, use outcomes to measure progress and adjust goals and interventions.

The first step should occur early in the intervention process. The selection of measures should be valid, reliable, and sensitive to changes in performance while aligning with the client's goals. The second step requires the occupational therapy practitioner to monitor progress toward the goal on an ongoing basis during the intervention. This provides data for decision making during the intervention review.

Evidence-Based Review of Interventions in Early Childhood

The following sections include both an overview of specific interventions and findings from the evidence-based literature of occupational therapy for young children ages birth through 5 years. A standard process of searching for and reviewing literature related to practice was used and is summarized in Appendix C. The research studies presented here include primarily *Level I* randomized controlled trials, systematic reviews, and meta-analyses; *Level II* studies, in which assignment to a treatment or a control group is not randomized

(cohort study); and *Level III* studies, which do not have a control group. In this systematic review, if Levels I, II, and III evidence for occupational therapy practice were adequate, then only those levels are used to answer a particular question.

All studies identified by the review, including those not specifically described in this section, are summarized and cited in full in the evidence tables in Appendix D. Readers are encouraged to read the full articles for more details.

Interventions Promoting Social–Emotional Development

A total of 23 articles were selected for appraisal in the systematic reviews of interventions used in occupational therapy to promote social–emotional development in children ages birth through 5 years. Social–emotional development is the ability of the child to self-soothe, regulate emotions, form relationships with others, and communicate their emotions (Zero To Three, 2010). Occupational therapists address social–emotional development through a variety of means, including improving a child's ability to self-regulate or providing direct instruction on appropriate social skills during activities taking place in the natural setting. The articles appraised are categorized into six themes: (1) touch-based intervention, (2) relationship-based interventions, (3) interactional/play-based activities to promote joint attention, (4) naturalistic intervention, (5) instruction-based intervention, and (6) therapist-selected toys and objects.

Touch-Based Intervention

Three articles related to the efficacy of touch-based intervention (Escalona et al., 2001; Tessier et al., 2003; von Knorring et al., 2008). Touch-based intervention included infant massage, massage techniques, and Kangaroo Care. Multiple studies supported the use of massage as a means of improving social–emotional development in a variety of populations of children.

Moderate evidence showed improvement in the areas of attention, restless and impulsive behavior, and decreased stereotypical behaviors in young children diagnosed with an ASD who received a 15-minute massage before bed (Escalona et al., 2001 [Level I]). In Swedish day care centers, the use of massage at daily rest time was shown to significantly improve aggressive and somatic problems in children identified as aggressive (von Knorring et al., 2008 [Level II]). Kangaroo Care, a method of holding an infant with skin-to-skin contact, was associated with moderate evidence that it promoted speech, eye–hand coordination, and social–emotional development in children born preterm (Tessier et al., 2003 [Level I]).

Relationship-Based Interventions

Five articles comprised this theme (Daunhauer, Coster, Tickle-Degnen, & Cermak, 2007; Field, Field, Sanders, & Nadel, 2001; Gutstein, Burgess, & Montfort, 2007; Mahoney & Perales, 2003, 2005). Studies within this theme described adult-directed play interactions, parent training in Responsive Teaching strategies, transactional intervention, and Relationship Development Intervention. Frequency of intervention, when reported, ranged from daily to weekly treatment, and duration ranged from 11 to 41 months.

Caregiver-facilitated play is moderately supported in the literature. In a Romanian orphanage, children demonstrated more developmentally competent play with a caregiver and were less anxious when caregivers were less anxious (Daunhauer et al., 2007 [Level II]). Parents who successfully used responsive teaching methods were associated with children demonstrating more attention, persistence, interest, cooperation, initiation, joint attention, affect, and social–emotional functioning at a low evidence level (Mahoney & Perales, 2003 [Level III]; Mahoney & Perales, 2005 [Level III]). Children who received Relationship Development Intervention showed statistically significant improvements on

the Autism Diagnostic Observation Schedule from pre- to posttesting (Gutstein et al., 2007 [Level III]). Occupational therapists should consider the incorporation of strategies derived from the various models described in this section to promote more developmentally competent play skills when working with children with developmental delays and those with an ASD.

Interactional/Play-Based Activities to Promote Joint Attention

A total of 4 articles were appraised that related to joint attention and adult–child interaction (Kasari, Freeman, & Paparella, 2006; Olafsen et al., 2006; Vismara, Colombi, & Rogers, 2009; Whalen, Schreibman, & Ingersoll, 2006). The interventions described under this theme included discrete trial, semistructured play sessions, joint attention, pivotal response training, the Early Denver Model, and the Vermont Intervention Program For Low Birth Weight Infants. The Early Denver Model consists of one-to-one interactions between an adult and child focused on turn-taking, the child's interests, and natural rewards. The Vermont Intervention Program For Low Birth Weight Infants consists of nursing visits in the hospital once a day for the 7 days prior to discharge and four home visits once the infant was discharged.

There is strong evidence suggesting that social initiation can be significantly improved for children born preterm and those with an ASD, through intervention (Kasari et al., 2006 [Level I]; Olafsen et al., 2006 [Level I]; Vismara et al., 2009 [Level IV]; Whalen et al., 2006 [Level IV]). Discrete trial combined with either semistructured play sessions or pivotal response training for children with ASD showed high levels of evidence of a positive impact on the acquisition of higher levels of structured play, although the studies found conflicting results related to improvements in symbolic play (Kasari et al., 2006; Whalen et al., 2006).

Naturalistic Interventions

Three articles in this systematic review related to naturalistic interventions to promote peer-to-peer engagement (Betz et al., 2008; Guralnick, Connor, Neville, & Hammond, 2006; Howard, Greyrose, Kehr, Espinosa, & Beckwith, 1996). Naturally occurring supports or treatments included photo-based activity schedules, scripts for adults and children, instructor-guided play, playgroups that included both children with and without disabilities, and instruction on computer use for developmentally appropriate activities. Evidence was inconclusive overall regarding dyad engagement from pre- to posttesting using visually scheduled and scripted instructor-guided play; however, 80% of measured change was sustained during the maintenance period (Betz et al., 2008 [Level IV]). The use of mixed playgroups for children with and without disabilities showed that both groups of children improved in their responsiveness to peers and total positive behavior; however, treatment conditions did not yield an impact (Guralnick et al., 2006 [Level I]). Instruction of preschool pairs in using the computer showed limited evidence of increased active waiting, turn-taking, and positive affect (Howard et al., 1996 [Level II]).

Instruction-Based Interventions

There were 6 articles analyzed under this theme (Crozier & Tincani, 2007; Hwang & Hughes, 2000; Kroeger, Schultz, & Newsom, 2007; Landa, Holman, O'Neill, & Stuart, 2011; Reichow & Volkmar, 2010; Vaughn et al., 2003). Interventions included Social Stories, direct teaching of social skills with video modeling, discrete trial training and pivotal response training, contingent imitation, natural reinforcement, environmental arrangement, applied behavior analysis therapy, prompting and rehearsal of target behaviors, play-related activities, modeling, storytelling, and reinforcement. Frequency and duration of interventions, when reported, ranged from 15 1-hr sessions to 10 hr a week with 38 hr of caregiver training.

Direct teaching with video modeling and applied behavioral analysis were associated with improved social skills with a high level of evidence in children with an ASD (Kroeger et al., 2007 [Level II]; Reichow & Volkmar, 2010 [Level I]). Pivotal response training and environmental arrangement had a high level of evidence supporting positive association with prolonging social interaction for children with an ASD (Hwang & Hughes, 2000 [Level I]; Landa et al., 2011 [Level I]). The use of Social Stories with children with an ASD was inconclusive in their effectiveness in reducing inappropriate behaviors and increasing appropriate behaviors (Crozier & Tincani, 2007 [Level IV]).

In their systematic review, Vaughn and colleagues (2003 [Level I]) found strong evidence that modeling, play-based activities, rehearsal of social behaviors, and prompting had a large effect size on positive social outcomes. Occupational therapists addressing social skills in early childhood should consider a combination of direct teaching, modeling, and pivotal response techniques both outside of and during play-based activities when working with children with an ASD.

Therapist-Selected Toys and Objects

There were 2 articles selected for appraisal under this theme (Kim et al., 2003 [Level I]; Tanta et al., 2005 [Level IV]). Interventions included manipulating the amount of space available during free play, therapist-modeled actions with toys, use of social and isolate toys, and free-play groups with peers matched with a peer with higher or lower play skills. Authors found moderate evidence that the use of social toys promoted cooperative play and positive social outcomes for children with disabilities in collaborative preschool classrooms (Kim et al., 2003). The use of mixed-level playgroups had moderately positive social outcomes for children with disabilities and children paired with peers with higher play skills (Kim et al., 2003; Tanta et al., 2005).

Interventions for Feeding, Eating, and Swallowing

A total of 34 articles were included in the evidence-based review of interventions for feeding, eating, and swallowing for children from birth through 5 years. AOTA (2007) defines *feeding* as "setting up, arranging, and bringing food [or fluid] from plate or cup to the mouth" (p. 26). *Eating* is described as "the ability to keep and manipulate food or fluid in the mouth and swallow it" (AOTA, 2007, p. 26). *Swallowing* is "a complicated act where food, fluid, medication, or saliva is moved from the mouth through the pharynx and esophagus to the stomach" (AOTA, 2007, p. 29).

Occupational therapy practitioners provide interventions to support feeding, eating, and swallowing through interventions targeted at improving the child's related performance skills. Three themes were identified based on the type of intervention used: (1) behavior-based interventions, (2) parent-directed/educational-based interventions, and (3) physiological-based interventions. The findings are presented in this section according to thematic analysis.

Behavioral-Based Interventions

Seven articles contributed to the behavioral-based intervention theme (Benoit et al., 2000; Byars et al., 2003; Greer et al., 2008; Kerwin, 1999; Laud et al., 2009; Wilder et al., 2005; Williams et al., 2007). Authors described various behavioral methods, including extinction, reinforcement, differential reinforcement, noncontingent reinforcement, token economies, and prompting. Often, the behavioral-based intervention studies contained elements of physiological intervention as well, including swallow induction, thermal stimulation, and oral–motor therapy. There is evidence to support the effectiveness of behavioral-based interventions to address a variety of feeding difficulties for children.

Behavioral interventions resulted in increased food acceptance during mealtimes for children with an ASD, autism, reflux, and food allergies (Laud et. al., 2009 [Level III]; Wilder et. al., 2005 [Level IV]). There was moderate evidence to support increased caloric intake as the result of behavioral interventions for children who are tube fed and resistant to oral feeding, tube dependent, liquid dependent, and food selective (Benoit et al., 2000 [Level I]; Greer et al., 2008 [Level III]; Williams et al., 2007 [Level III]). Two articles reported children being successfully weaned from tube feedings by means of behavioral interventions with low levels of evidence strength (Byars et al., 2003 [Level III]; Williams et al., 2007 [Level III]). The evidence supports the use of behavioral interventions in conjunction with physiological interventions to target a variety of feeding outcomes.

Parent-Directed or Educational-Based Interventions

This theme included 6 articles (Black et al., 1995; Chatoor, Hirsch, & Persinger, 1997; Fraser et al., 2004; Garcia Coll et al., 1996; Pinelli, Atkinson, & Saigal, 2001; Pridham et al., 2005). Parent-directed or educational-based interventions included home-based intervention, parent education programs, video-based training, guided participation with home visits and phone calls, and individual counseling. The evidence suggests that parent-directed and educational-based interventions are effective in addressing child and parent outcomes.

There was moderate evidence that an individualized behavioral feeding intervention was effective in increasing physical growth of infants (Black et al., 1995 [Level I]; Chatoor et al., 1997 [Level III]; Garcia Coll et al., 1996 [Level I]). There is limited evidence suggesting that parent education and parent-directed intervention reduce maternal stress (Chatoor et al., 1997 [Level III]; Pridham et al., 2005 [Level I]). Authors also found limited evidence that these interventions improved mealtime behaviors and reduced problem eating (Fraser et al., 2004 [Level III]). Overall, using parent-directed intervention in the home was supported as beneficial to infants and young children with feeding difficulties. It is important to note that there is research suggesting that overall quality of life may be improved for families secondary to the reduction in maternal stress.

Physiological-Based Interventions

A total of 21 articles in this systematic review related to physiological interventions (S. M. Barlow, Finan, Lee, & Chu, 2008; Bier et al., 1996; Boiron, Da Nobrega, Roux, Henrot, & Saliba, 2007; Bragelien, Rokke, & Markestad, 2007; Einarsson-Backes, Deitz, Price, Glass, & Hays, 1994; Fucile, Gisel, & Lau, 2002, 2005; Gaebler & Hanzlik, 1996; Gisel et al., 2003; Hake-Brooks & Anderson, 2008; Jadcherla et al., 2009; Lamm, De Felice, & Cargan, 2005; Larnert & Ekberg, 1995; Moore, Anderson, & Bergman, 2007; Munakata et al., 2008; Pinelli & Symington, 2005; Poore, Zimmerman, Barlow, Wang, & Gu, 2008; Reid, 2004; Rocha, Moreira, Pimenta, Ramos, & Lucena, 2007; Simpson, Schanler, & Lau, 2002; White-Traut et al., 2002). Interventions included skin-to-skin contact, an oral support and stimulation multidisciplinary intervention, positioning, nonnutritive sucking, sensory motor–oral stimulation, oral feeding, multisensory intervention, NTrainer System scenting, and Vojta's technique to initiate reflex activity. Vojta's technique is a therapeutic strategy based on locomotion reflexes. The NTrainer System is an electronic pacifier that measures and improves infant sucking and pre-feeding oral–motor skills. Frequency of described interventions varied from single to multiple times in a day.

There was strong evidence that oral stimulation programs significantly affect nonnutritive sucking pressure and the quantity of milk ingested during oral feeding (Boiron et al., 2007 [Level I]; Fucile et al., 2005 [Level I]; Pinelli & Symington, 2005 [Level I]). There was moderate evidence that tactile and multisensory interventions significantly improve nipple feeding in pre-term infants, neonates with dysphagia, and pre-term infants

with and without central nervous system injuries (Gaebler & Hanzlik, 1996 [Level II]; Jadcherla et al., 2009 [Level III]; White-Traut et al., 2002 [Level I]). There is strong evidence that the use of oral stimulation programs, skin-to-skin contact, and sensory motor–oral interventions result in shortened length of stays in both pre-term infants and full-term healthy infants (Fucile et al., 2002 [Level I]; Moore et al., 2007 [Level I]; Rocha et al., 2007 [Level I]). Several studies support the use of physiological interventions, including oral stimulation interventions, early introduction of oral feeding, and Vojta's technique, for successful transition from tube to oral feeding in infants born pre-term (Bragelien et al., 2007; Fucile et al., 2002, 2005; Simpson et al., 2002). Many articles reported a variety of isolated outcomes that were not confirmed by other articles within this review.

Overall, physiological interventions led to improved sucking pressure, oral intake during feedings, nipple feeding, and discontinuation of tube feedings. The evidence suggests that behavioral, parent-directed, and physiological interventions are effective in addressing feeding difficulties in young children who were born pre-term and/ or have a history of tube feeding. Occupational therapists may want to use a combination of these interventions when addressing feeding, eating, and swallowing difficulties in children.

Interventions for Improving Cognitive Development

A total of 13 studies met the inclusion criteria for the evidence-based review of effective interventions for improving cognitive development in children from birth to age 5. Cognitive development in children involves the acquisition of skills related to perception, memory, language, concepts, and problem solving (AOTA, 2008). Occupational therapy practitioners support cognitive development through their use of interventions and activities facilitating the development of attention, visual perception, memory, concepts, and problem solving. Themes related to the location of intervention emerged and include NICU, home, and natural environments. Another theme was related to the use of interventions to promote joint attention.

NICU Interventions

Two studies examined interventions that took place in the NICU (Kleberg, Westrup, Stjernqvist, & Lagercrantz, 2002; Maguire et al., 2009). Two studies examined the use of the NIDCAP, a program designed to provide individual care to promote enhanced interactions between parents and infants through careful observations and adjustments to the levels of stimulation the infant is exposed to. Kleberg and colleagues (2002 [Level I]) found that the infants in the NIDCAP treatment group had significantly higher cognitive development, as measured by the Bayley Scales of Infant Development (Bayley, 1993), than the control group infants. In their follow-up study, Maguire and colleagues (2009 [Level I]) did not find statistically significant lasting differences at 1- and 2-year follow-up points. Therefore, evidence supporting the use of NIDCAP is inconclusive at this time.

NICU-to-Home Interventions

Four articles discussed interventions initiated in the NICU, which had a component that extended into the home (Barrera, Kitching, Cunningham, Douchet, & Rosenbaum, 1991; Melnyk et al., 2001; Nelson et al., 2001; Orton, Spittle, Doyle, Anderson, & Boyd, 2009). All articles provided overall moderate evidence supporting home-based interventions.

Barrera and colleagues (1991 [Level I]) compared two different in-home treatment conditions with a control group. They did not find any significant results for the differing interventions; however, low-birthweight infants in the control group were found to be lower performing than all other groups. Melnyk and colleagues (2001 [Level I]) examined the use of Creating Opportunities for Parent Empowerment program, which educates mothers about physical characteristics and behaviors of their low-birthweight infant, how to interact with their infant, and activities to promote development. Infants who participated in the Creating Opportunities for Parent Empowerment group showed significantly higher cognitive scores at both 3 and 6 months' corrected age according to the Bayley Scales of Infant Development. It was found that infants treated using a multisensory approach that addressed auditory, tactile, visual, and vestibular inputs in the hospital through 2 months' corrected age had higher motor and mental performance indicators than controls (Nelson et al., 2001 [Level I]). Orton and colleagues (2009 [Level I]) examined an early intervention program that focused on cognitive and motor outcomes for pre-term infants and found short-term cognitive gains in infancy and preschool.

Interventions Promoting Joint Attention

Four articles examined the use of interventions to increase joint attention in children who were born pre-term, were low birthweight, and were diagnosed with autism (Gulsrud, Kasari, Freeman, & Paparella, 2007; Olafsen et al., 2006; Whalen et al., 2006; Wong, Kasari, Freeman, & Paparella, 2007). Interventions included methods such as discrete trial training, pivotal response training, applied behavioral analysis, and joint attention and symbolic play activities. In their comparison of intervention focused on either joint attention or symbolic play, Gulsrud and colleagues (2007 [Level I]) found moderate evidence that children with autism in the joint attention intervention group improved in acknowledgment of novel objects and maintained coordinated looks for a longer period of time.

Similarly, Wong and colleagues (2007 [Level I]) examined joint attention intervention against symbolic play incorporating applied behavior analysis in preschool children with autism. Their results were inconclusive; however, they reported that children on the autism spectrum mastered criteria during table-based activities before generalizing to floor play.

In their randomized control trial, Olafesen and colleagues (2006 [Level I]) followed up on an early intervention program for low-birthweight infants that was initiated in the NICU then continued into the home for four home visits after discharge. At the 12-month follow-up, there was moderate evidence demonstrating that the treatment group scored significantly higher on initiating joint attention, initiating object requests, and responding to social interaction (Olafsen et al., 2006 [Level I]).

Whalen and colleagues (2006 [Level II]) found that typically developing children and children with autism in a treatment group using discrete trial training and pivotal response training when addressing joint attention improved in social initiation, spontaneous speech, and play skills. The sample size was very small during this cohort study; therefore, the strength of this evidence is limited and should be interpreted with caution.

Interventions to Promote Motor Development

In the evidence-based review of interventions to promote motor development, 24 articles were selected for appraisal. Several themes emerged in the literature: (1) developmental interventions for at-risk infants, (2) interventions for young children at risk for CP, and (3) visual–motor interventions for preschool children with developmental delays. Occupational therapy practitioners may target motor development through their use of neurodevelopmental treatment, biomechanical intervention, practice of motor tasks, sensory-based interventions, and constraint-induced movement therapy (CIMT).

Developmental Interventions for At-Risk Infants

There were 5 articles that discussed the use of developmental interventions for at-risk infants, including children at high risk for developmental disabilities; pre-term infants born before 37 weeks with neuromuscular diagnosis and those with developmental disabilities; pre-term infants born after 37 weeks; and typically developing children (Blauw-Hospers & Hadders-Algra, 2005; Chiarello & Palisano, 1998; Lekskulchai & Cole, 2001; McManus & Kotelchuck, 2007; Orton et al., 2009). Interventions included sensory stimulation, motor intervention strategies, parent–infant interaction strategies, caregiver-delivered home programs, aquatic therapy, parent education, and behavioral intervention therapy. The findings across articles were mixed.

In their systematic review, Blauw-Hospers and Hadders-Algra (2005 [Level I]) reported improvement in 13 out of 34 studies and no improvement with interventions (i.e., sensory stimulation, neurodevelopmental treatment, NIDCAP) applied after the neonatal period. Orton and colleagues (2009 [Level I]) found that although early intervention improved cognitive outcomes, it had a limited impact on motor outcomes based on several measures, including the Test of Infant Motor Performance (Campbell et al., 2002), the Bayley Scales of Infant Development (Bayley, 1993), and the Griffiths Mental Development Locomotor subscale (Griffiths, 1996). McManus and Kotelchuck (2007 [Level III]) found that aquatic therapy in addition to home-based early intervention improved functional mobility; however, the results were not statistically significant.

Moderate evidence supported infants who received a caregiver-delivered home program that was updated at 1, 2, and 3 months made significant improvements on the Test of Infant Motor Performance compared to controls (Lekskulchai & Cole, 2001 [Level I]). Chiarello and Palisano (1998 [Level I]) examined the impact of a 5-wk parent education program that modeled appropriate activities to promote fine and gross motor skill development, at the conclusion of which the treatment and the control groups were not different.

Interventions for Young Children With or at Risk for Cerebral Palsy

There were 15 articles that discussed interventions for children with or at risk for CP (Aarts, Jongerius, Geerdink, van Limbeek, & Guerts, 2010, 2011; Arndt, Chandler, Sweeney, Sharkey, & McElroy, 2008; Brown & Burns, 2001; Catanese, Coleman, King, & Reddihough, 1995; DeLuca, Echols, Law, & Ramey, 2006; Girolami & Campbell, 1994; Law et al., 1991, 1997, 2011; Mayo, 1991; Reddihough, King, Coleman, & Catanese, 1998; Sakzewski, Ziviani, & Boyd, 2009; Taub, Ramey, DeLuca, & Echols, 2004; Willis, Morello, Davie, Rice, & Bennett, 2002). Interventions examined by the authors included CIMT, neurodevelopmental treatment (NDT), conductive education, child-focused intervention, and context-focused intervention. Populations of children in the studies included infants with posture and movement dysfunction, children from ages 1 year to 7 years diagnosed with CP, pre-term infants, children with hemiplegia, and children with hemiparesis.

Several studies that examined CIMT found positive results and strong evidence supporting its use for young children diagnosed with CP and hemiplegia. In their meta-analysis of NDT, CIMT, habit training, and Botox injections, Sakzewski and colleagues (2009 [Level I]) found positive outcomes associated with CIMT. Willis and colleagues (2002 [Level I]) also found a significant increase in children's use of their hemiparetic upper extremity after CIMT by casting the unimpaired arm for 1 month. Two additional studies found improved motor function in children with CP from 14 to 86 months of age who underwent casting of their unimpaired upper extremities for 21 days compared to controls (DeLuca et al., 2006 [Level I]; Taub et al., 2004 [Level I]). Law and colleagues

(1991 [Level I]) found that adding casting to an intensive NDT program improved the quality of movement; however, the results were not statistically significant and therefore inconclusive.

Aarts and colleagues (2010 [Level I]) completed two studies that examined modified CIMT, which included bimanual task training. The first study found statistically significant improvements for children in the modified CIMT group compared to controls. In a secondary analysis of their 2010 data, Aarts and colleagues (2011 [Level I]) found the quality and frequency of use improved in the upper extremity with spasticity, but strength and automaticity did not improve.

Many studies examined the use of NDT, with mixed results. In their systematic review, Brown and Burns (2001 [Level I]) found inconsistent evidence supporting NDT as an effective treatment for children with neurodysfunction based on measures including the Peabody Developmental Motor Scales, goniometry, and the Bayley Scales of Infant Development. Law and colleagues (1991 [Level I]) found no significant differences between groups randomly assigned to intensive NDT with casting, regular NDT with casting, intensive NDT, and regular NDT intervention groups based on their scores on Peabody Developmental Motor Scales Fine Motor Scales. They did note improved quality of movement for the intensive NDT and casting group using the Quality of Upper Extremity Skills Test; however, the results were not statistically significant. In a later study, Law and colleagues (1997 [Level II]) compared NDT and casting and found no significant difference between groups.

When comparing basic NDT (monthly) to intensive NDT (weekly) for 6 months, Mayo (1991 [Level I]) found statistically significant improved outcomes for the intensive group in their aggregate scores for motor development. Arndt and colleagues (2008 [Level II]) compared NDT to a parent–infant play protocol and found children who received the NDT made significantly greater gains in their gross motor function. Overall, the studies were inconclusive regarding the use of NDT to improve motor outcomes for children with CP.

Five studies examined conductive education (CE) as an intervention (Blank, von Kries, Hesse, & von Voss, 2008; Catanese et al., 1995; Coleman, King, & Reddihough, 1995; Hur, 1997; Reddihough et al., 1998). CE originated in Hungary and uses a master conductor to lead children in social units to perform activities designed to improve their control of functional movements (Reddihough et al., 1998 [Level I]). Blank and colleagues (2008 [Level III]) found that the CE group made statistically significant improvement compared to the group receiving special education with weekly therapy in their hand functions and ADLs in children 3 to 6 years old with CP.

In the first study conducted by Catanese and colleagues (1995 [Level II]), the authors compared CE with individual physiotherapy and found improvement in both groups, but the children in CE made greater improvements in fine motor skills, gross motor skills, and ADLs. Later, the same team of authors compared individual therapy and CE to NDT and playgroups with caregivers (Reddihough et al., 1998 [Level I]). They found the group with CE and individual therapy made greater gains in cognition, but there was not a significant difference between groups for gross motor skill improvement. In their study comparing CE to care as usual early intervention over a 26-week period, Coleman and colleagues (1995 [Level II]) found no statistically significant results. Similarly, Hur (1997 [Level II]) did not find any statistically significant in skills comparing 3½- to 4½-year-old children receiving CE or special education services. Interestingly, Hur found that the CE group sustained adverse impact in hip function.

Overall, the evidence for CE is inconclusive. In a recent study, Law and colleagues (2011 [Level I]) looked at child-focused versus context-focused intervention in 128 children with CP over 6 months. Both approaches were equally effective, and there were no significant differences between the groups.

Visual–Motor Interventions for Children With Developmental Delays

Four studies examined visual–motor interventions for young children with developmental delays (Case-Smith, 2000b; Dankert et al., 2003; Davies & Gavin, 1994; DeGangi, Wietlisbach, Goodin, & Scheiner, 1993). DeGangi and colleagues (1993 [Level II]) compared therapist-directed sensorimotor therapy to child-directed sensorimotor therapy and found that therapist-led therapy promoted improved gross motor and functional skills, whereas child-led therapy promoted improved fine motor skills. Children who received occupational therapy and had developmental delays made significant improvement from pre- to posttesting as assessed by the Beery–Buktenica Developmental Test of Visual Motor Integration (Dankert et al., 2003 [Level II]).

Davies and Gavin (1994 [Level II]) compared 10 children who received direct occupational and physical therapy weekly to 8 children who received weekly consultation from occupational and physical therapists with classroom staff and found that both groups improved in fine and gross motor skills based on the Peabody Developmental Motor Scales (2nd ed. Folio & Fewell, 2000), and there were no significant differences between groups. Case-Smith (2000a [Level III]) found that preschoolers who received occupational therapy made statistically significant improvements in manipulation, motor accuracy, fine motor skills, and visual–motor skills. In addition, Case-Smith concluded that sessions, including peer interaction and play, were related to visual–motor skill improvement. In general, there is limited evidence supporting the use of visual–motor interventions.

Service Delivery in Early Childhood

In total, 42 articles related to service delivery in early childhood were reviewed. Of these articles,

18 met inclusion criteria. The included studies clustered around several themes or perspectives. The themes used to categorize interventions from the review included home, community, and natural settings; routines; and parent training/parent–child relationship.

Setting

Five articles described intervention results based on the setting in which the service was provided, for example, a home-based, center-based, or community-based setting (Bierman et al., 2008; Bruder, 1997; Chazan-Cohen et al., 2007; Love et al. 2005; Luiselli, O'Malley-Cannon, Ellis, & Sisson, 2000). Bierman and colleagues (2008 [Level I]) found moderate evidence that supports that the use of a combined setting approach across classroom and home environments led to improved outcomes in executive functioning for children attending Head Start programs. Further supporting the use of a combination of environments, Bruder (1997 [Level II]) found that services at an early intervention center, in a group environment, and using a consultative model were correlated with greater motor and social change than the alternatives. A mix of both center- and home-based intervention was found to have the greatest impact on child cognitive and language development, child social–emotional development, and parenting behavior (Love et al. 2005 [Level I]). On the basis of the articles reviewed, there is moderate evidence supporting that occupational therapists should use approaches across environments and settings.

Duration of intervention is another area examined in the literature. Luiselli and colleagues (2000 [Level II]) found duration of treatment (number of months) was a statistically significant predictor of change for children diagnosed with autism or pervasive developmental disorder participating in a home-based behavioral intervention. Chazan-Cohen and colleagues (2007 [Level I]) found moderate evidence showing a greater impact on maternal depression when the children began Early Head Start at age 2 years than children who began Early Head Start at age 3. The research suggests that intervening earlier in a child's life may have greater impact.

Routines

Many studies analyzed routine-based or contextualized interventions and, overall, the evidence found was limited. A study conducted by Bruder (2003 [Level II]) found significant improvements in both affect and engagement in children identified as English-language learners treated weekly during high-interest activities over 24 weeks. Dunst and colleagues (2006 [Level II]) showed that the more intervention took place during the everyday learning opportunities, the more positive the consequences for perceived parental control, parenting competence, positive parent well-being, and parent's judgment of child progress for children receiving early intervention services. The use of contextualized intervention was further supported by Moes and Frea (2002 [Level III]), who found that intervention that took place during family routines led to extinguished target behaviors and generalization of skills. Occupational therapists should consider observing and developing interventions to support the child's and the family's occupations and activities, including home programs, during naturally occurring routines and learning opportunities within a family's schedule.

Several studies supported the use of family-centered intervention. *Family-centered help-giving* is the philosophy and practice of incorporating the values and choices of families and providing support to strengthen the family. Dunst, Trivette, and Hamby (2007 [Level I]) found moderate evidence that family-centered help-giving had significant positive results on self-efficacy beliefs, participant satisfaction, parenting behavior, personal and family well-being, social support, and child behavior. While studying the effectiveness of a family-based model of intervention, McCart, Wolf,

Sweeney, and Chai (2009 [Level II]) did not find statistically significant results for their model; however, parents reported less stress as a direct result of their participation in the model. Romer and Umbreit (1998 [Level III]) found that families rated services that used family-centered service delivery as more important, and 76% of families were highly satisfied with family-centered service delivery. The literature suggests improved attainment of parental outcomes with the use of family-centered intervention models.

Parent Training/Parent–Child Relationship

Articles in this theme discussed results in terms of parent outcomes, child outcomes, and parent satisfaction. J. Barlow, Coren, and Stewart-Brown (2009 [Level I systematic review]) addressed whether group-based parenting programs were effective in improving maternal psychosocial health. They found statistically significant results, with strong evidence favoring the intervention group for decreased depression, anxiety, and stress; increased self-esteem; and improved relationships with spouse/marital adjustment. VanLeit and Crowe (2002 [Level I]) found statistically significant increases in satisfaction scores on the Canadian Occupational Performance Measure for mothers of children with disabilities attending an 8-week group program. The literature suggests that group parenting interventions are effective for parent-based outcomes.

In a study conducted by Chang, Park, and Kim (2009 [Level I]), the results showed moderate evidence of increased cognitive scores in children whose parents attended Early Head Start parenting classes compared to children in the control group. Lakes and colleagues (2009 [Level IV]) examined a community-based group parenting program and found significant improvements in overall child difficulty and conduct problems, as well as high levels of satisfaction with the program. The same study found offering supports to families such as meals, flexible scheduling, and child care improved program attendance.

In an examination of media-based behavioral interventions (i.e., computer-, video-, or audio-based programs), Montgomery, Bjornstad, and Dennis (2009 [Level I]) found that child behavioral outcomes were significantly improved with the addition of 2 hours of therapist time versus just the media-based intervention. Media-based interventions included booklets, DVDs, cassettes, and computer programs. The literature suggests overall moderate evidence strength supporting group parent training as effective in producing positive outcomes for children.

Whitaker (2002 [Level III]) found that parent training to support child development in the areas of communication, play, and behavior was highly valued by parents. A study conducted by Hume, Bellini, and Pratt (2005 [Level IV]) found that parents highly rated parent training, sensory integration therapy, and self-contained classrooms. The highest level of correlation found in the study was between the use of regular progress reports and perceived quality-of-life outcomes. These findings further support the use of parent training and family-centered intervention.

Summary and Implications for Occupational Therapy Practice

The Systematic Reviews of Early Childhood included a total of 112 appraised articles. Of the total, 65 were Level I articles, 18 were Level II articles, 17 were Level III articles, and 12 were Level IV articles. Level V articles were excluded from this review. More than half the articles were at the highest level of evidence. All the articles selected for appraisal can be found in the evidence tables located in Appendix D.

Practitioners are encouraged to read the full articles for complete details and understanding of the individual studies. Practitioners also are encouraged to read the recommendations presented in Table 10, which are based on the evidence presented in the systematic reviews.

There are many factors to consider when applying the evidence from the literature to practice. It is recommended that the practitioner be mindful of the level and strength of the evidence, limitations of the studies, clinical expertise, client preferences, and any factors that may affect generalization of the findings to a population presenting in the practitioner's clinical setting.

Implications for Practice

In many studies, combinations of interventions, rather than individual interventions, were used. For example, when addressing feeding, physiological and behavioral interventions often were combined (Byars et al., 2003; Williams et al., 2007); when addressing upper extremity use in children with CP, NDT and CIMT often were used together (Law et al., 1991, 1997); and in addressing social skills, video modeling was paired with direct teaching methods (Kroeger et al., 2007). In some studies, researchers controlled for various combinations of interventions, and others did not. It will be important for practitioners to use caution in interpreting the efficacy of an intervention in isolation that was paired with another intervention in a study.

Social–Emotional Development

Sensory interventions were effective in promoting physiological stability in infants. Instruction and tools such as Social Stories, visual schedules, toys with sensory components, modeling, and contingent reinforcement were associated with promoting social behaviors and peer interaction (Gutstein et al., 2007; Kasari et al., 2006; Mahoney & Perales, 2005; Vaughn et al., 2003). The social competence of preschool-age children developed with peer-mediated strategies and direct instruction. Coaching parents to improve their interaction and understanding of their children can promote joint attention, cooperation, initiation, and positive affect in their children (Olafsen et al., 2006; Vismara et al., 2009).

Occupational therapy practitioners should consider the following to promote social behaviors, joint attention, and peer interaction:
- Incorporate typical peers and coach parents to improve joint attention when working with children with an ASD
- Structure group sessions that use visual supports, contingent reinforcement, modeling, and direct instruction.

Table 10. Recommendations for Occupational Therapy Intervention for Early Childhood: Birth Through 5 Years

Interventions	Recommended	No Recommendation	Not Recommended
Social–Emotional			
Touch-based interventions			
	Infant massage to improve sleep and relaxation, reduce crying, and reduce hormones affecting stress, but no change for cognitive and behavioral outcomes (A)		
	Massage before bed to improve attention, reduce restless and impulsive behavior, and decrease stereotypical behaviors in young children (B)		
	Kangaroo Care to promote social–emotional development, eye–hand coordination, and speech (B)		
Relationship-based intervention			
	Caregiver-facilitated play to reduce anxiety in children and parents and to increase developmentally competent play (B)		
	Use of responsive teaching methods by parents to increase attention, persistence, interest, cooperation, initiation, joint attention, affect, and social–emotional functioning (C)		
Interactional/play-based activities			
	Discrete trial combined with either semistructured play sessions or pivotal response training to improve structured play (A)		
	Discrete trial combined with either semistructured play sessions or pivotal response training to improve symbolic play (I)		
Naturalistic interventions			
	Mixed play groups (children with and without disabilities) to improve responsiveness to peers and improve total positive behavior for both groups (B)		
	Instruction of preschool pairs in using a computer to increase active waiting, turn-taking, and positive affect (C)		
	Visually scheduled and scripted instructor-guided play to improve dyad engagement (I)		
Instruction-based intervention			
	Modeling, play-based activities, rehearsal of social behaviors, and prompting to improve social behaviors (A)		

(Continued)

Table 10. Recommendations for Occupational Therapy Intervention for Early Childhood: Birth Through 5 Years *(Cont.)*

Interventions	Recommended	No Recommendation	Not Recommended
	Direct teaching with video modeling and applied behavior analysis to improve social skills (A)		
	Pivotal response training and environmental arrangement to prolong social interaction (A)		
	Social Stories to reduce inappropriate behaviors and increase appropriate behaviors (I)		
Therapist-selected toys and objects			
	Use of social toys to promote cooperative play and positive social outcomes (B)		
	Mixed-level play groups for children with disabilities and children paired with peers with better play skills to improve social outcomes (B)		
Feeding, Eating, and Swallowing			
Behavioral-based interventions			
	Use of behavioral interventions to increase calorie intake (B)		
	Use of behavioral interventions to wean from tube feedings (C)		
Parent-directed educational-based interventions			
	Use of individualized behavioral feeding intervention to increase physical growth of infants (B)		
	Parent education and parent-directed intervention reduces maternal stress (B)		
	Use of behavioral interventions to increase food acceptance during mealtimes (C)		
	Parent education and parent-directed intervention to improve mealtime behaviors and reduce problem behaviors (C)		
Physiological interventions			
	Oral stimulation programs to increase nonnutritive sucking pressure and the quantity of milk ingested during oral feeding (A)		
	Oral stimulation programs, skin-to-skin contact, and sensory–motor–oral interventions to reduce the length of hospital stay (A)		

(Continued)

Table 10. Recommendations for Occupational Therapy Intervention for Early Childhood: Birth Through 5 Years *(Cont.)*

Interventions	Recommended	No Recommendation	Not Recommended
	Tactile and multisensory interventions to improve nipple feeding (B)		
	Oral stimulation, early introduction of oral feeding, and Votja's techniques to improve transition from tube to oral feeding (I)		
Cognitive Interventions			
Neonatal intensive care unit (NICU)			
	Use of Newborn Individualized Developmental Care and Assessment Program to improve infant cognitive development (I)		
NICU and home-based interventions			
	A multisensory approach addressing auditory, tactile, visual, and vestibular input in the hospital and at home until 2 months' corrected age to improve mental and motor performance (B)		
	Use of a parent education program that includes information on behavior, interaction with infants, and activities to promote development (B)		
	An early intervention program for preterm infants to improve cognitive outcomes in infancy and preschool (B)		
Intervention to promote joint attention			
	Intervention incorporating joint attention to improve maintenance of coordinated looks and with increased acknowledgment of novel objects (B)		
	Early intervention program started in hospital and continued with home visits to improve joint attention and initiating object requests (B)		
	Discrete trial training and pivotal response training when addressing joint attention to improve social limitations, spontaneous speech, and play skills (C)		
	Outcomes comparing the use of joint attention interventions vs. interventions using symbolic play and applied behavioral analysis were inconclusive (I)		

(Continued)

Table 10. Recommendations for Occupational Therapy Intervention for Early Childhood: Birth Through 5 Years *(Cont.)*

Interventions	Recommended	No Recommendation	Not Recommended
Interventions to Promote Motor Performance			
Developmental interventions for at-risk infants			
	A caregiver-delivered home program for infants updated at 1, 2, and 3 months to improve motor performance (B)	5-week long parent education that models appropriate motor development (I)	
	Developmental motor interventions to improve motor outcomes (I)		
Interventions for children with or at risk for cerebral palsy (CP)			
	Use of constraint-induced movement therapy to improve motor performance in young children with CP (A)	Conductive education to improve motor performance in young children with CP (I)	
	Use of neurodevelopmental treatment for young children with CP to improve motor performance (I)		
	Child-focused and context-focused intervention were equally likely to improve motor performance (B)		
Visual–motor interventions for children with developmental delays			
	Therapist-led sensorimotor therapy to improve gross motor and functional skills. (C)		
	Child-led sensorimotor therapy to improve fine motor skills (C)		
	Occupational therapy for preschoolers to improve visual–motor and fine motor skills, manipulation, and motor accuracy (C)		
	Direct or indirect occupational therapy were equally likely to improve visual motor skills (C)		
Service Delivery in Early Childhood			
Studies regarding setting			
	Providing interventions at more than one setting (e.g., classroom and home) to improve performance outcomes (B)		
	Participation in a Head Start Program at age 2 rather than age 3 to reduce maternal depression (B)		
	Longer duration of home-based behavioral treatment to improve outcomes of children with autism or pervasive developmental disorder (C)		

(Continued)

Table 10. Recommendations for Occupational Therapy Intervention for Early Childhood: Birth Through 5 Years *(Cont.)*

Interventions	Recommended	No Recommendation	Not Recommended
Studies regarding routine-based intervention			
	Family-centered help-giving that incorporates support to strengthen the family to improve satisfaction, parenting behavior, personal and family well-being, social support, and child behavior (B)		
	Use of routines-based or contextualized interventions to improve affect and engagement (C)		
	Use of everyday learning opportunities to improve parenting competence, parental well-being, and parent's judgment of child progress (C)		
	Interventions taking place during family routines to extinguish target behaviors and improve generalization of skills (C)		
	Family-centered service delivery to improve satisfaction and reduce family stress (C)		
Studies regarding parent training			
	Parenting programs to improve parent-based outcomes (e.g., parent stress, anxiety, depression) (A)		
	Early Head Start parenting classes to improve cognitive outcomes in early childhood (B)		
	Addition of brief therapist-led parenting education to improve behavioral outcomes of young children (B)		
	Parent training to improve satisfaction and quality of life (C)		
	Community-based parenting group to reduce child difficulty and conduct problems (I)		

Note. Criteria for level of evidence (A, B, C, I, D) are based on standard language from the Agency for Healthcare Research and Quality (2009). Suggested recommendations are based on the available evidence and content experts' clinical expertise regarding the value of using the intervention in practice. A = There is strong evidence that occupational therapy practitioners should routinely provide the intervention to eligible clients. Good evidence was found that the intervention improves important outcomes and concludes that beneëts substantially outweigh harm. B = There is moderate evidence that occupational therapy practitioners should routinely provide the intervention to eligible clients. At least fair evidence was found that the intervention improves important outcomes and concludes that beneëts outweigh harm. C = There is weak evidence that the intervention can improve outcomes, and the balance of the beneëts and harms may result either in a recommendation that occupational therapy practitioners routinely provide the intervention to eligible clients or in no recommendation as the balance of the beneëts and harm is too close to justify a general recommendation. I = Insufécient evidence to determine whether or not occupational therapy practitioners should be routinely providing the intervention. Evidence that the intervention is effective is lacking, of poor quality, or conñicting and the balance of beneëts and harm cannot be determined. D = Recommend that occupational therapy practitioners do not provide the intervention to eligible clients. At least fair evidence was found that the intervention is ineffective or that harm outweighs beneëts.

Feeding, Eating, and Swallowing

Feeding interventions can be implemented by occupational therapists or caregivers trained and monitored by an occupational therapist. It is important to match the intervention appropriately to the underlying difficulty affecting a client's occupational performance. For example, the use of a behavioral approach to intervention was most successful for mealtime behaviors, acceptance of food, and oral intake, whereas physiological interventions were most appropriate for children with neuromuscular impairments or with abnormalities with their oral structures (Benoit et al., 2000; Byars et al., 2003; Greer et al., 2008; Kerwin, 1999; Laud et al., 2009). Parent-directed interventions were effective when the goals of intervention were to improve maternal outcomes, parenting outcomes, and mother–child interaction (Black et al., 1995; Pridham et al., 2005). Interdisciplinary behavioral interventions were effective in both inpatient and outpatient settings (Benoit et al., 2000; Byars et al., 2003; Kerwin, 1999).

When addressing feeding, eating, and swallowing, occupational therapy practitioners should consider

- Incorporating behavioral approaches to increase food acceptance, oral intake, and to decrease inappropriate mealtime behaviors
- Using physiological interventions for children with atypical oral structures or those neuromuscular impairments.

Cognitive Development

Interventions originating in the NICU and that provided a component extending into the home improved cognitive outcomes for pre-term infants (Nelson et al., 2001; Orton et al., 2009). Inconclusive results were found for the use of the NIDCAP program in the NICU for cognitive outcomes (Kleberg et al., 2002; Maguire et al., 2009). Preschool-age children diagnosed with an ASD made gains in joint attention when behavioral interventions targeting joint attention were paired with child-directed play (Whalen et al., 2006; Wong et al., 2007).

In their support of cognitive development occupational therapy, practitioners should

- Incorporate behavior strategies and child-led play when working with children with an ASD who need to improve in the area of joint attention
- Use interventions across home, community, and school environments.

Motor Performance

Interventions that incorporated social elements, play, collaboration with the family, and functional outcomes resulted in improved functional performance for children in early childhood (Aarts et al., 2010; Case-Smith, 2000a; DeLuca et al., 2006; Law et al., 2011; McManus & Kotelchuck, 2007; Reddihough et al., 1998). Studies that examined outcomes for at-risk infants found mixed results (Blauw-Hospers & Hadders-Algra, 2005; Chiarello & Palisano, 1998; Lekskulchai & Cole, 2001; McManus & Kotelchuck, 2007; Orton et al., 2009). Overall, the evidence on motor outcomes for at-risk infants is inconclusive. Consultation and direct intervention were found to be equally effective in addressing gross motor, fine motor, and visual–motor outcomes for preschool children; however, the studies were of lower level evidence (Case-Smith, 2000a; Davies & Gavin, 1994; Law et al., 2011).

Occupational therapy practitioners working to improve motor performance may consider

- Incorporating play and collaboration with the family to improve outcomes
- Carefully considering the use of direct treatment versus consultation.

Service Delivery

Embedding intervention in the natural routines of a family led to positive outcomes as measured by parent report of the efficacy of and satisfaction with an intervention. Parenting programs show positive results for a variety of family outcomes, child outcomes, and familial relationships (Barlow et al., 2009; Hume et al., 2005; Whitaker, 2002). The literature suggests that interventions implemented across multiple environments were more effective than interventions that took place in a singular environment (Bruder, 1997; Chazan-Cohen et al., 2007; Love et al., 2005).

When making decisions regarding service delivery, occupational therapy interventionists should consider
- Embedding intervention within the naturally occurring routines of the family
- Implementing intervention across the multiple environments or contexts for the child.

Implications for Research

Additional research based on stronger study designs is needed to determine the effectiveness of interventions used by occupational therapy practitioners with children from birth through 5 years. Participation by occupational therapy researchers in interdisciplinary research programs would enhance the development of evidence for interventions to support feeding, eating, swallowing, social–emotional development, motor development, and cognitive development. In the areas of caregiver training and implementation of intervention, more research is needed specific to fathers and nontraditional families. Beyond types of intervention, research is needed to examine the impact of variables associated with service delivery, such as setting or context of intervention, frequency of intervention, consultation versus direct intervention, and duration of the intervention.

Implications for Education

Educational programs for occupational therapy practitioners should adhere to the educational standards of their national accrediting body. On the basis of the systematic reviews, some implications for inclusion and/or emphasis of content have been revealed. Encouraging and supporting translational research for the field of occupational therapy is important to adequately respond to gaps in professional literature related specifically to occupational therapy practice. Providing strategies on how to best embed interventions into a family's or a classroom's naturally occurring routines should be emphasized in educational programs (Barlow et al., 2009; Hume et al., 2005; Whitaker, 2002). Increasing student knowledge and application of behavioral approaches would support improved outcomes related to both feeding and social emotional outcomes (Benoit et al., 2000; Byars et al., 2003; Kerwin, 1999; Whalen et al., 2006; Wong et al., 2007).

Implications for Policy

Occupational therapy practitioners are key members of interdisciplinary teams that provide interventions during early childhood. It would be advantageous for occupational therapy practitioners to have a presence in policymaking that reflects their level of involvement with children during the early childhood years. This would include assuming positions on local, state, and national public service and political organizations that influence policy for children from birth through 5 years. However, more information regarding the impacts of specific factors, such as setting, service delivery model, and frequency and duration of services would be helpful to guide professional advocacy regarding funding and legislation.

Appendix A. Preparation and Qualifications of Occupational Therapists and Occupational Therapy Assistants

Who Are Occupational Therapists?

To practice as an occupational therapist, the individual trained in the United States

- Has graduated from an occupational therapy program accredited by the Accreditation Council for Occupational Therapy Education (ACOTE®) or predecessor organizations;
- Has successfully completed a period of supervised fieldwork experience required by the recognized educational institution where the applicant met the academic requirements of an educational program for occupational therapists that is accredited by ACOTE or predecessor organizations;
- Has passed a nationally recognized entry-level examination for occupational therapists; and
- Fulfills state requirements for licensure, certification, or registration.

Educational Programs for the Occupational Therapist

These include the following:
- Biological, physical, social, and behavioral sciences

- Basic tenets of occupational therapy
- Occupational therapy theoretical perspectives
- Screening evaluation
- Formulation and implementation of an intervention plan
- Context of service delivery
- Management of occupational therapy services (master's level)
- Leadership and management (doctoral level)
- Professional ethics, values, and responsibilities.

The fieldwork component of the program is designed to develop competent, entry-level, generalist occupational therapists by providing experience with a variety of clients across the lifespan and in a variety of settings. Fieldwork is integral to the program's curriculum design and includes an in-depth experience in delivering occupational therapy services to clients, focusing on the application of purposeful and meaningful occupation and/or research, administration, and management of occupational therapy services. The fieldwork experience is designed to promote clinical reasoning and reflective practice, to transmit the values and beliefs that enable ethical practice, and to develop professionalism and competence in career responsibilities. Doctoral-level students also must complete a doctoral experiential component designed to develop advanced skills beyond a generalist level.

Who Are Occupational Therapy Assistants?

To practice as an occupational therapy assistant, the individual trained in the United States

- Has graduated from an occupational therapy assistant program accredited by ACOTE or predecessor organizations;
- Has successfully completed a period of supervised fieldwork experience required by the recognized educational institution where the applicant met the academic requirements of an educational program for occupational therapy assistants that is accredited by ACOTE or predecessor organizations;
- Has passed a nationally recognized entry-level examination for occupational therapy assistants; and
- Fulfills state requirements for licensure, certification, or registration.

Educational Programs for the Occupational Therapy Assistant

These include the following:

- Biological, physical, social, and behavioral sciences
- Basic tenets of occupational therapy

- Screening and assessment
- Intervention and implementation
- Context of service delivery
- Assistance in management of occupational therapy services
- Professional ethics, values, and responsibilities.

The fieldwork component of the program is designed to develop competent, entry-level, generalist occupational therapy assistants by providing experience with a variety of clients across the lifespan and in a variety of settings. Fieldwork is integral to the program's curriculum design and includes an in-depth experience in delivering occupational therapy services to clients, focusing on the application of purposeful and meaningful occupation. The fieldwork experience is designed to promote clinical reasoning appropriate to the occupational therapy assistant role, to transmit the values and beliefs that enable ethical practice, and to develop professionalism and competence in career responsibilities.

Regulation of Occupational Therapy Practice

All occupational therapists and occupational therapy assistants must practice under federal and state law. Currently, 50 states, the District of Columbia, Puerto Rico, and Guam have enacted laws regulating the practice of occupational therapy.

Note. The majority of this information is taken from the *2011 Accreditation Council for Occupational Therapy Education (ACOTE) Standards* (ACOTE, 2012).

Appendix B.
Selected *Current Procedural Terminology*™ (*CPT*) Codes for Occupational Therapy Evaluations and Interventions for Young Children (Birth–5 Years)

The following chart may assist occupational therapists in making clinically appropriate decisions in selecting the most relevant *CPT* code to describe occupational therapy evaluation and intervention for young children. Occupational therapy practitioners should use the most appropriate code from the current *CPT* manual based on specific services provided, individual patient goals, payer coding and billing policy, and common usage.

Examples of Occupational Therapy Evaluation and Intervention	Suggested *CPT* Code(s)
Evaluation	
Initial evaluation of the young child's performance in areas of occupation, performance skills, performance patterns, context and environment, activity demands, and client factors. • Functional evaluation using standardized and nonstandardized assessments and gathering of data from various other sources (e.g., medical record, occupational profile, interview, caregivers, significant others). • Develop occupational therapy treatment plan, including individual goals to address performance deficits.	97003—Occupational therapy evaluation

(Continued)

Examples of Occupational Therapy Evaluation and Intervention	Suggested *CPT* Code(s)
Formal reassessment of changes in performance due to changes in status, diagnosis, or if intervention plans needs significant revisions. • Reassessment of young child's status and progress, using standardized and nonstandardized assessments as well as other data sources (interviews with caregivers, significant others, physicians).	97004—Occupational therapy reevaluation
Administer and interpret results of standardized assessments of neurocognition, including global cognitive functions, executive function, memory, learning, problem solving, constructional praxis, language, attention, and other neural substrates for occupational performance.	96125—Standardized cognitive performance testing per hour of a qualified health care professional's time, both face-to-face time administering tests to the patient and time interpreting these test results and preparing the report
Administer measurement to assess physical performance skills in children.	97750—Physical performance test or measurement (e.g., musculo-skeletal) with written report, each 15 minutes
Administer, interpret, and report findings from assistive technology assessment to identify technology to improve a young child's performance and participation.	97755—Assistive technology assessment (e.g. to restore, augment or compensate for existing function, optimize functional tasks and/or maximize environmental accessibility), direct one-on-one contact by provider, with written report, each 15 minutes
Participate in a medical team conference as part of a diagnostic/evaluation team whereby the team discusses with a client's family the evaluation findings, diagnoses, and recommendations.	99366—Medical team conference with interdisciplinary team of health care professionals, face-to-face with patient and/or family, 30 minutes or more, participation by nonphysician qualified health care professional
Participate in a medical team conference as part of a diagnostic/evaluation team whereby the team reviews evaluation findings and clarifies diagnostic considerations and recommendations prior to meeting with a client's family.	99368—Medical team conference with interdisciplinary team of health care professionals, patient and/or family not present, 30 minutes or more; participation by nonphysician qualified health care professional
Intervention	
Provide exercises to increase strength, endurance, range of motion, flexibility, and mobility to enhance ability to participate in daily activities.	97110—Therapeutic procedure, one or more areas, each 15 minutes; therapeutic exercises to develop strength and endurance, range of motion and flexibility
Design and implement graded activities to increase coordination, balance, and sensory awareness to enhance participation in daily occupations. • Application of techniques to promote adaptive responses to sitting, standing, and posturing to facilitate participation in desired occupation after a stroke (brain bleed). • Develop and train in use of motor responses to effect change in functional performance (e.g., toileting, dressing).	97112—Therapeutic procedure, one or more areas, each 15 minutes; neuromuscular reeducation of movement, balance, coordination, kinesthetic sense, posture, and/or proprioception for sitting and/or standing activities

(Continued)

Examples of Occupational Therapy Evaluation and Intervention	Suggested *CPT* Code(s)
Design and train in aquatic exercise program to improve functioning. Train family in aquatic exercise program to be completed at home or a local pool. • Direct group activities for 2 or more clients to support a common goal • Group intervention focusing on fine motor activities or social interactions.	**97113**—Therapeutic procedure, one or more areas, each 15 minutes; aquatic therapy with therapeutic exercises **97150**—Therapeutic procedure(s), group (2 or more individuals; report 97150 for each member of group); group therapy procedures involve constant attendance of the physician or therapist but by definition do not require one-on-one patient contact by the provider (use of dynamic activities to improve functional performance), each 15 minutes
Design and implement a variety of individual therapeutic activities to facilitate the child's participation and performance at home and in the community. This may include • Games and puzzles to enhance visual motor processing so child can play with family and friends • Working on self-care skills so child is more independent.	**97530**—Therapeutic activities, direct (one-on-one) patient contact by the provider (use of dynamic activities to improve functional performance), each 15 minutes
Individualized intervention focusing on improvement of cognitive skills. Train family in the use of strategies to enhance child's problem-solving skills.	**97532**—Development of cognitive skills to improve attention, memory, problem solving (includes compensatory training), direct (one-on-one) patient contact by the provider, each 15 minutes
Design and implement occupational therapy interventions using sensory integration techniques to facilitate adaptive responding and optimal arousal to allow for enhanced participation in play, school, and adaptive occupations.	**97533**—Sensory integrative techniques to enhance sensory processing and promote adaptive responses to environmental demands, direct on-on-one patient contact by the provider, each 15 minutes
Provide instruction to improve participation and performance in adaptive/self-care activities, including training family in methods of feeding, dressing, or positioning young child.	**97535**—Self-care/home management training (e.g., activities of daily living (ADL) and compensatory training, meal preparation, safety procedures, and instructions in use of assistive technology devices/adaptive equipment), direct one-on-one contact by provider, each 15 minutes
Assess and fit a young child with a hand splint for a beginning hand contracture.	**97760**—Orthotic(s) management and training (including assessment and fitting when not otherwise reported), upper extremity(s), lower extremity(s) and/or trunk, each 15 minutes

Note. Medical team conferences are not billable to Medicare; however, these codes may be useful for reporting productivity. The *CPT* 2013 codes referenced in this document do not represent all of the possible codes that may be used in occupational therapy evaluation and intervention. Not all payers will reimburse for all codes. Refer to *CPT* 2013 for the complete list of available codes. *CPT* is a trademark of the American Medical Association. All rights reserved. Codes shown refer to *CPT* 2013. *CPT* codes are updated annually. New and revised codes become effective January 1. Always refer to annual updated *CPT* publication for most current codes.

Appendix C.
Evidence-Based Practice

Since 1998, the American Occupational Therapy Association (AOTA) has instituted a series of evidence-based practice (EBP) projects to assist members with meeting the challenge of finding and reviewing the literature to identify evidence and, in turn, using this evidence to inform practice (Lieberman & Scheer, 2002). Following the evidence-based philosophy of Sackett, Rosenberg, Muir Gray, Haynes, and Richardson (1996), AOTA's projects are based on the principle that the EBPs of occupational therapy rely on the integration of information from three sources: (1) clinical experience and reasoning, (2) preferences of clients and their families, and (3) findings from the best available research.

A major focus of AOTA's EBP projects is an ongoing program of systematic review of multidisciplinary scientific literature, using focused questions and standardized procedures to identify practice-relevant evidence and discuss its implications for practice, education, and research. Systematic reviews of early intervention and early childhood research strengthen current knowledge of the efficacy of practices used by occupational therapy practitioners in services for young children.

An evidence-based perspective is founded on the assumption that scientific evidence of the effectiveness of occupational therapy intervention can be judged to be more or less strong and valid according to a hierarchy of research designs, an assessment of the quality of the research, or both. AOTA uses standards of evidence modeled on those developed in evidence-based medicine. This model standardizes and ranks the value of scientific evidence for biomedical practice using the grading system presented in Table C.1.

This study was initiated and supported by AOTA as part of the Evidence-Based Practice Project. In 2007, a Representative Assembly (RA) motion was passed "to charge the President to direct the Executive Director to direct resources to conduct an evidence-based literature review on the effectiveness of Occupational Therapy Services and Early Intervention." The RA charge reflected the need for occupational therapy practitioners to access findings from systematic reviews to support interventions within the scope of occupational therapy practice. In addition, the rationale for the RA charge was the increased incidence of childhood disorders and an interest in addressing barriers to early intervention occupational therapy services.

Four focused questions were initially developed for the systematic reviews of occupational therapy interventions for early intervention/early childhood and included questions related to social–emotional development; feeding, eating, and swallowing; preliteracy; and service delivery models. The questions were generated in conjunction with a group of content experts in early intervention/early childhood and EBP. Because of budget constraints, the project was put on hold until 2009. Following the review of the results of the search and development of summaries of the literature, the preliteracy question was divided into two questions, one examining intervention effects on motor outcomes

Table C.1. Levels of Evidence for Occupational Therapy Outcomes Research

Evidence Level	Definition
I	Systematic reviews, meta-analyses, randomized controlled trials
II	Two groups, nonrandomized studies (e.g., cohort, case control)
III	One group, nonrandomized (e.g., before and after, pretest and posttest)
IV	Descriptive studies that include analysis of outcomes (e.g., single-subject design, case series)
V	Case reports and expert opinion that include narrative literature reviews and consensus statements

Note. From "Evidence-Based Medicine: What It Is and What It Isn't," by D. L. Sackett, W. M. Rosenberg, J. A. Muir Gray, R. B. Haynes, and W. S. Richardson, 1996, *British Medical Journal, 312,* pp. 71–72. Copyright © 1996 by the British Medical Association. Adapted with permission.

and the other examining interventions that promote cognitive development related to preliteracy.

The following five focused questions from the review of interventions for children 0 through 5 years were included in this Practice Guideline:

1. *Social–emotional development*: What is the effectiveness for interventions used in occupational therapy to promote social–emotional development for children 0 through 5?
2. *Feeding, eating, and swallowing*: What is the evidence for the effectiveness for interventions used in occupational therapy to improve feeding, eating, and swallowing for children 0 through 5?
3. *Motor development*: What is the evidence for the effectiveness of interventions within the scope of occupational therapy to improve motor performance for children 0 through 5?
4. *Cognitive development*: What is the evidence for the effectiveness of interventions within the scope of occupational therapy practice to improve cognitive development for children 0 through 5?
5. *Service delivery model*: What is the evidence for the effectiveness of different service delivery models used to improve occupational performance for children 0 through 5 and families receiving early intervention and early childhood services?

Methodology

Search terms for the reviews were developed by the consultant to the AOTA Evidence-Based Practice Project and AOTA staff in consultation with the authors of each question and reviewed by the advisory group. The search terms were developed not only to capture pertinent articles but also to make sure that the terms relevant to the specific thesaurus of each database were included. Table C.2 lists the search terms related to the population and interventions included in each systematic review. A medical research librarian with experience in completing systematic review searches conducted all searches and confirmed and improved the search strategies.

Databases and sites searched included Medline, PsycINFO, CINAHL, Educational Resources Information Center (ERIC), and OTseeker. In addition, consolidated information sources, such as the Cochrane Database of Systematic Reviews and the Campbell Collaboration, were included in the search. These databases are peer-reviewed summaries of journal articles and provide a system for clinicians and scientists to conduct evidence-based reviews of selected clinical questions and topics. Moreover, reference lists from articles included in the systematic reviews were examined for potential articles, and selected journals were hand-searched to ensure that all appropriate articles were included.

Table C.2. Search Terms for Systematic Reviews for Early Childhood

Category	Key Search Terms
Population	Infant development, infant (newborn), infant (premature), infants, preschool children, toddlers, young children.
Intervention—Social emotional development	Affective attunement, attachment, attachment behavior, developmentally supportive care, coping, coping skills, DIR/Floortime, early childhood development (can include neonatal and infant development), early childhood play behavior, emotional development, family-centered care, family relations, individualized developmental care, infant care, infant massage, infant mental health, kangaroo care, mental health, mother–child relations, neonatal development, NIDCAP, occupational therapy, parent training, parental support, parent–child relations, parenting, parenting skills, pivot training, play, relationship-based interventions, routines-based interventions, self-regulation, sensorimotor/sensory motor, sensorimotor/sensory motor development, sensory integration, sensory integrative, social–emotional, synactive model of infant behavior.
Intervention—Feeding, eating, swallowing	Bottle feeding, breast feeding, breast feeding positions, caregiver/infant interaction during feeding, chewing, cup drinking, dysphagia, eating behavior, feeding, feeding and eating disorders of childhood (Medline), feeding difficulties, feeding habits, feeding problems, feeding readiness, finger feeding, food refusal, food textures, infants; nutrition, infant nutritional physiological phenomena (Medline), lactation, mealtime routines, mealtimes, non-nutritive sucking, oral feeding, oral sensorimotor, oral motor stimulation, oral support, pre-feeding oral stimulation, positioning during feeding, seating, suck, sucking/swallowing coordination, swallowing.
Intervention—Service delivery models	Activities-based, at-risk children, coaching, center-based, consultation, deficit model, developmentally appropriate practices, direct service, distributed learning, early childhood education, ecocultural model, ecocultural theory, ecological model, family centered, home visiting, home visits, iatrogenic effects, inclusion, inclusion (combined with preschool), integrated model, interdisciplinary, monitoring, natural environments, natural learning environment, NICU follow-up, parent-centered, parent family adaptation, routines based, service coordination, service delivery, strengths based, transdisciplinary, transdisciplinary teaming.
Intervention—Motor and cognitive	Activities of daily living, adaptive equipment, alphabet exposure, alphabet principle, assistive technology, attention, auditory processing, childhood play behavior, cognitive processing, computer games, computers, early childhood intervention, early intervention, early literacy, fine motor, fine motor skill learning, games, gross motor, gross motor skill learning, hand skills, handwriting, haptic perception/training, imitative behavior, imitation skills, joint attention, kinesthetic perception/training, language, manipulation skills, motor activity, motor processes, name writing, nonverbal, occupational therapy, perceptual learning, perceptual motor learning, perceptual motor processes, phoneme, phonemic awareness, physical development, play, play and playthings, postural balance, postural control, posture, pre-emergent writing, print awareness, problem solving, psychomotor, psychomotor performance, reading, rhythm, self-care, sensation, sensory integration, sensory processing, shared reading, skill learning, shoulder control, signing, sign language, sound awareness, space perception, spatial ability, transition, visual motor, visual perception, visual perceptual skills, visual spatial ability, Wii.

Inclusion and exclusion criteria are critical to the systematic review process because they provide the structure for the quality, type, and years of publication of the literature incorporated into a review. The review of all five questions was limited to peer-reviewed scientific literature published in English. The review also included consolidated information sources such as the Cochrane Collaboration. Reports listed on ERIC were included for the service delivery question.

The literature included in the review had been published between 1990 and 2010, and the study samples were children birth to age 5 and eligible for early intervention services. The intervention approaches examined were within the scope of practice of occupational therapy. The review excluded data from presentations, conference proceedings, non-peer-reviewed research literature, dissertations, and theses. Studies included in the review are Level I, II, and III evidence. Level IV evidence was included only where higher level evidence on a given topic was not found.

A total of 10,676 citations and abstracts were included in the reviews. The question on social–emotional development had 5,823 references; the feeding, eating, and swallowing question resulted in 1,147; the service delivery model question had 500; and the motor and cognitive questions yielded 3,206 citations and abstracts. The consultant to the EBP Project completed the first step of eliminating references based on citation and abstract. Except in one situation in which the author worked on the review independently, the reviews were carried out as academic partnerships in which academic faculty worked with graduate students. Review teams completed the next step of eliminating references based on citations and abstracts. The full-text versions of potential articles were retrieved, and the review teams determined final inclusion in the review based on predetermined inclusion and exclusion criteria.

A total of 112 articles were included in the final review. Table C.3 presents the number and levels of evidence for articles included in each review question. The teams working on each focused question reviewed the articles according to their quality (scientific rigor and lack of bias) and levels of evidence. Each article included in the review was then abstracted using an evidence table that provides a summary of the methods and findings of the article and an appraisal of the strengths and weaknesses of the study based on design and methodology. AOTA staff and an EBP Project consultant reviewed the evidence tables to ensure quality control.

The strength of the evidence is based on the guidelines of the U.S. Preventive Services Task Force (http://www.uspreventiveservicestaskforce.org/uspstf/grades.htm). The designation of "strong evidence" includes consistent results from well-conducted studies, usually at least two randomized controlled trials. A designation of "moderate evidence" may be based on one randomized controlled trial or two or more studies of lower levels of evidence. In addition, there may be some inconsistency of findings across individual studies that might preclude a classification of strong evidence. The designation of "limited evidence" may be based on few studies, flaws in the available studies, and some inconsistency in the findings across individual studies. A designation of "mixed" may indicate that the findings were inconsistent across studies in a given category. A designation of "insufficient evidence" may indicate that the number and quality of studies is too limited to make any clear classification.

Table C.3. Number of Articles in Each Review at Each Level of Evidence

Review	Evidence Level					Total in Each Review
	I	II	III	IV	V	
Social–emotional development	11	4	3	5	0	23
Feeding, eating, and swallowing	18	3	10	3	0	34
Service delivery models	8	4	3	3	0	18
Motor development	16	7	1	0	0	24
Cognitive development	12	0	0	1	0	13
Total	65	18	17	12	0	112

Review authors also completed a Critically Appraised Topic, a summary and appraisal of the key findings, clinical bottom line, and implications for occupational therapy based on the articles included in the review for each question.

Strengths and Limitations of the Systematic Reviews

The five systematic reviews presented in this Practice Guideline have several strengths and include many aspects of occupational therapy practice for infants, toddlers, young children, and their families. The reviews included 112 articles, and three-fourths of the articles were Level I and II evidence, indicating that the evidence was of high quality. The reviews also involved systematic methodologies and incorporated quality control measures.

The limitations of the systematic reviews are based on the design and methods of individual studies and include small sample sizes and limited descriptions of the psychometric properties of a study's outcome measures. In addition, many of the studies in the review included concurrent interventions, and separating the effects of a single intervention may be difficult.

Appendix D.
Evidence Tables

Table D.1. Evidence for Social–Emotional Development Interventions

Author/Year	Study Objectives	Level/Design/Participants	Intervention and Outcome Measures	Results	Study Limitations
Touch-Based Interventions					
Escalona et al. (2001)	To examine the effect of parent-administered massage therapy on behavior in children with autism	Level 1—Randomized control trial. N = 20 children with ASD (12 boys, 8 girls) ages 3–6 yr Mean age = 5.2 yr, SD = 1.8	*Intervention* *Massage therapy:* The parents provided massage therapy for 15 min before bedtime every night for 1 mo. *Control group:* The parents read a Dr. Seuss story. *Outcome Measures:* • Revised Conners Scales for ADHD • Behavior observations in the classroom and on the playground • Sleep diaries.	The children with massage improved on impulsive behavior and inattentiveness when preintervention and postintervention scores were compared. Children showed a decrease in stereotypical behaviors and an increase in on-task behavior. Sleep problems improved.	Short-term study with no follow-up.
http://dx.doi.org/10.1023/A:1012273110194					
Tessier et al. (2003)	To examine the effect of kangaroo mother care (KMC) on infants' mental development	Level 1—Randomized control trial. Initially included 431 low-birth-weight, preterm infants, all < 1,801 g, at 12 mo; 336 mother–infant dyads *KMC group:* 183 dyads (Mean gestational age = 33 wk, birthweight = 1,536 g) *Traditional care group:* 153 dyads (Mean gestational age = 33 wk, birth weight = 1,565 g)	*Intervention* KMC was provided continuously until the infant was 37–38 wk gestation age (using different care providers). *Outcome Measures* • The Griffiths test of cognitive development administered at 12 mo IQ • INFANIB (infant neurological assessment), used to measure neurological integrity.	Using IQ scores, KMC infants were 3.7 points higher than traditional care infants at 12 mo, a significant difference. The areas that showed the greatest effect were speech, performance (eye–hand skills), and personal social skills. Skin-to-skin contact may promote bonding and emotional development. KMC may promote cortical organization at a critical time of infant development.	Lack of information about the infants' experiences in the year after KMC. Limited information about the participants.
http://dx.doi.org/10.1016/S0163-6383(03)00037-7					

Study	Study Objectives	Level/Design/Participants	Intervention and Outcome Measures	Results	Study Limitations
von Knorring et al. (2008)	To evaluate the effects of massage in 4- to 5-yr-old children with aggression and deviant behavior	Level II—Nonrandomized, two groups. *N* = 110 children (53 boys, 57 girls), typically developing Massage group *n* = 60 Control group *n* = 50 Age range 4–5 yr	*Intervention* *Massage group:* Massage consisting of slow stroking and kneading during the rest period at Swedish day care centers. *Control group:* Listened to stories. *Outcome Measure* Swedish translation of the Child Behavior Checklist (CBCL).	When the massage and control groups were compared after 6 mo of intervention, children who were rated higher on the CBCL (i.e., demonstrated more aggressive behaviors) showed decreases in aggressive behavior and somatic problems.	Limited applicability to occupational therapists.

http://dx.doi.org/10.1111/j.1651-2227.2008.00919.x

Relationship-Focused Interventions

Study	Study Objectives	Level/Design/Participants	Intervention and Outcome Measures	Results	Study Limitations
Daunhauer et al. (2007)	To investigate whether institutionalized children demonstrate more developmentally competent play when interacting with a caregiver than when playing alone and to identify what type of interaction is most associated with competent play	Level II—Two groups, nonrandomized study. *N* = 26 children in a Romanian orphanage (Mean age = 10.3 mo, Mean developmental age = 9 mo) Mean duration of residence in orphanage = 14.6 mo (range = 10–38 mo) 11 caregivers from the orphanage participated (Mean age = 33 yr).	*Intervention* The caregivers interacted with the children in play using a set of exploratory toys and a set of pretend toys. *Each child participated in two 6-min independent play sessions and one session with a known caregiver.* *Outcome Measures* • Caregiver Interaction Rating Scale, selected items, to evaluate play interaction • Developmental Play Scale to evaluate developmental play Measured by students. Reliability was evaluated.	The institutionalized children demonstrated significantly more developmentally competent play when interacting with a caregiver (*d = 0.53*). Children with lower cognition or longer institutionalization benefited less. Children were less anxious when the caregiver was less anxious. Children were more successful when the caregiver assisted, directed, and structured the task and when the caregiver was encouraging and warm.	Limited generalizability to U.S. populations. Low sample size.

http://dx.doi.org/10.5014/ajot.61.4.429

(Continued)

Table D.1. Evidence for Social–Emotional Development Interventions *(Cont.)*

Author/Year	Study Objectives	Level/Design/Participants	Intervention and Outcome Measures	Results	Study Limitations
Field et al. (2001)	To determine whether multiple sessions of an adult imitating the behavior of children with autism increases their social initiations and responsiveness	Level I—Randomized control trial. *Participants* N = 20 children with autism, nonverbal (10 girls, 10 boys) Mean age = 5.4 yr	*Intervention* After random assignment, a 4-phase procedure was used. In the 1st phase, an adult sat with a still face; then the adult either imitated all of the child's behaviors or was contingently responsive to the child's behaviors. In the 3rd phase, the adult returned to a still face. The 4th phase was spontaneous play interaction. *Outcome Measures* The children's behavior was videotaped, and trained coders rated social behaviors and play behaviors every second for 3 min.	The children who received imitation showed less time being inactive or playing alone; more time showing object behaviors (accepting and playing with objects); more time looking at the adult, vocalizing to the adult, and smiling at the adult; and more time showing imitation recognition and engaging in reciprocal play.	Measured immediate effects of a few sessions; effects over time unknown.

http://dx.doi.org/10.1177/1362361301005003008

Author/Year	Study Objectives	Level/Design/Participants	Intervention and Outcome Measures	Results	Study Limitations
Gutstein et al. (2007)	To evaluate the effectiveness of relationship development intervention (RDI) in a sample of children with ASD on their autism symptoms	Level III—One group, nonrandomized, pretest–posttest. *Participants* N = 16 children with ASD; 8 with secondary diagnosis of language disorder, 5 with bipolar disorder, 1 with ADHD, and 1 with food allergies; 15 boys, 1 girl Age range = 21–94 mo	*Intervention* Children were in RDI an average of 41.5 mo. The parents were trained in a 6-day workshop. They met with the therapists for weekly or biweekly consultation to update the program plan and to review videotaped segments of the parent and child working on the program. The parents learned how to perceive and scaffold opportunities for their child to respond in a flexible way to challenging events. *Outcome Measures* • Autism Diagnostic Interview–Revised (ADI–R) • Autism Diagnostic Observation Schedule (ADOS), a measure of parental perception of their child's flexibility and adaptation • Evaluation of school placement.	The children in the RDI group demonstrated significantly greater improvement on the ADOS from pre- to posttest. 70% of children in the RDI group improved. The change on the ADI–R was significant. Children rated as flexible went from 16% to 71%. At follow-up, 31% of children were in special education settings, compared with 86% before intervention.	No control group. No blinded evaluation. Small sample size.

Mahoney & Perales (2003)	To investigate the effectiveness of relationship-focused intervention on the social and emotional well-being of children with ASD and whether these effects relate to parents' responsiveness	Level III—One group, pretest–posttest. *N* = 20 children with ASD (12 boys, 8 girls), all with cognitive delay and problems in social–emotional skills Mean age = 32 mo (*SD* = 7.1)	*Intervention* Length of intervention was 31 sessions over 11.4 mo. Trained therapists met with parent and child each week to help parents learn responsive teaching strategies. These meetings helped parents learn responsive interactive behaviors: reciprocity, contingency, shared control, affect, and match. *Outcome Measures* • Temperament and Atypical Behavior Scales, which measures parents' perception of child's temperament and behavior • Infant Toddler Social Emotional Assessment, which assesses internalizing, externalizing, and regulatory problems • Child Behavior Rating Scale • Maternal Behavior Rating Scale, which assesses parent–child interaction.	Mothers made significant gains in using responsiveness and affect (increased 35% and 27%) and did not change in achievement orientation and directiveness (declined 13% and 4%). Children showed 50% higher ratings in attention, persistence, interest, cooperation, initiation, joint attention, and affect. Changes in maternal responsiveness accounted for 25% of the variance in changes in children's social interactive behavior.	No control group. Small sample size. No blinded evaluation.

http://dx.doi.org/10.1177/02711214030230020301

Mahoney & Perales (2005)	To compare the effects of relationship-focused early intervention on young children with ASD with those on children with developmental disabilities	Level III—Nonrandomized, two groups, each of which received the same treatment. *N* = 50 young children with either ASD or other developmental disability (DD) *n* = 20 children with ASD, 13 children with DD, 14 children with speech and language delay, and 3 children categorized as "other" Mean age = 26.4 mo, range = 12–54 mo	*Intervention* Teaching mothers to become more responsive to their children. In this model, the effects of responsive interaction strategies on children's development are mediated by the impact that they have on pivotal developmental behaviors. Treatment was provided weekly for 1-hr sessions, for approximately 1 yr. *Outcome Measures* • Transdisciplinary Play Based Assessment, a child development profile • Infant Toddler Social Emotional Assessment • Temperament and Atypical Behavior Scale • Child Behavior Rating Scale, which measures pivotal developmental behavior • Maternal Behavior Rating Scale (MBRS), which measures parent interaction.	Mothers made significant increases in responsiveness as measured by the MBRS. Children made gains in development and social–emotional functioning; Rates of development changed from 20% to 259%. Children with ASD improved more on the developmental measures than children with DD. Changes in mothers' responsiveness accounted for 20% of the variance in changes in children's pivotal developmental behavior.	No control group. No blinded evaluation.

http://dx.doi.org/10.1097/00004703-200504000-00002

(Continued)

Table D.1. Evidence for Social–Emotional Development Interventions *(Cont.)*

Author/Year	Study Objectives	Level/Design/Participants	Intervention and Outcome Measures	Results	Study Limitations
Olafsen et al. (2006)	To evaluate the effects of optimized neonatal mother–infant transactions on joint attention at 12 mo and to analyze whether an early intervention program to increase parents' sensitivity to infants' behaviors enhances joint attention at 12 mo	Level I—Randomized control trial. *N* = 140 preterm infants, 75 term infants Intervention group, *n* = 71 (36 boys, 35 girls); Mean gestational age = 30 wk Control group, *n* = 69 (37 boys, 32 girls); Mean gestational age = 30 wk Term infants, *n* = 75 (40 boys, 35 girls); Mean gestational age = 39 wk	*Intervention* The Vermont Intervention Program for Low Birth Weight Infants (Rauh Achenbach, Nurcombe, Howell, & Teti, 1988), which emphasizes transition: parents appreciating their baby's specific behaviors and being sensitive to the infant's cues and teaching parents to respond to cues. Neonatal nurses met with the parents every day for 7 days before discharge. They made 4 home visits after discharge. *Outcome Measures* • The Early Social Communication Scales • Joint attention behaviors, behavioral requests, and social interaction behaviors were measured through behavioral counts from videotaped sessions.	The preterm intervention group was significantly higher in initiating joint attention and responding to social interaction. The term group scored moderately higher than the preterm control group. The infants did not show differences in responding to joint attention or responding to requests. Children's ability to integrate complex information may not be affected by this intervention.	Limited applicability to occupational therapists. Limited description of the intervention in the report.

http://dx.doi.org/10.1016/j.infbeh.2006.07.004

Joint Attention Interventions

Kasari et al. (2006)	To examine the efficacy of interventions targeting joint attention and symbolic play on these skills in children with ASD	Level I—RCT with two conditions and one control. *N* = 58 children with ASD Joint attention group, *n* = 20; Mean age = 43.2 mo (*SD* = 7.1) Play group, *n* = 21; Mean age = 42.7 mo (*SD* = 6.9) Control group, *n* = 17 in the control; Mean age = 42.9 mo (*SD* = 4.9)	*Intervention* Each child received 5–8 min of discrete trial on a new goal, then the child worked on that goal in a semistructured, child-centered play session. This session targeted symbolic play or joint attention. *Outcome Measures* • Early Social Communication Scales • Structured Play Assessment (play level) • Caregiver–child interaction.	Compared with the control group, children in the joint attention group improved more in responding to joint attention. Children in the play group showed more diversity of play and higher play levels. Effect sizes were large, and the children generalized their new skills to different contexts.	Appeared to have overlap in the two conditions: joint attention and symbolic play.

http://dx.doi.org/10.1111/j.1469-7610.2005.01567.x

Landa et al. (2011)	To evaluate the effect of supplementing a comprehensive intervention with a curriculum targeting socially synchronous behavior (interpersonal synchrony) on social outcomes in toddlers with ASD	Level I—Randomized control trial. $N = 48$ toddlers with ASD (age 21–33 mo), matched on receptive language, social interaction Interpersonal synchrony (IS) condition: $n = 24$ (20 boys, 4 girls); Mean age = 28.6 mo ($SD = 2.6$) Noninterpersonal synchrony (NIS) condition: $n = 24$ (20 boys, 4 girls); Mean age = 28.8 mo ($SD = 2.8$)	*Intervention* For 10 hr/wk, intervention directly targeted the development of socially engaged imitation, joint attention, and affect sharing. Both groups received classroom-based intervention for 196–205 hr, using discrete trial teaching, pivotal response training, and visual communication systems. 38 hr of parent education were included. *Outcome Measures* • Initiation of joint attention and shared positive affect were measured using the Communication and Symbolic Behavior Scales Developmental Profile • Socially Engaged Imitation as defined by eye contact was rated from videotapes.	The children who receive the IS intervention improved more in social engaged interaction; initiation of joint attention and shared positive affect were no different between groups. The IS group showed a large effect for initiation of joint attention (d = 0.86–1.56). Both groups made significant gains in social, cognitive, and language skills.	Children receiving additional interventions were not described.
http://dx.doi.org/10.1111/j.1469-7610.2010.02288.x				
Vismara et al. (2009)	To pilot a brief, time-limited manualized intervention for parent education using the Early Start Denver Model	Level IV—Multiple baseline, single subject. $N = 8$ children (initially 10, 2 dropped out), 7 of whom had a diagnosis of ASD; 1 had symptoms consistent with ASD Age range = 10 mo–3 yr	*Intervention* The Early Denver Model includes 1:1 interactions between therapist and child or parent and child. The strategies are: increase child's attention; sensory social routines; dyadic engagement; nonverbal communication; imitation; joint attention; speech development; antecedent–behavior–consequence; prompting, shaping, fading; functional assessment. *Outcome Measures* • Social communication and social engagement in 10-min samples of child–parent play • Child Behavior Rating Scale • Parent's fidelity of implementation.	Parents correctly implemented the early start techniques with 93%–97% accuracy. Children's production of functional verbal responses increased; child engagement, attentiveness, and social initiative behaviors increased. A 12-wk intervention can be effective with young children at risk for ASD. The intervention was effective with 2 children who had aggressive, disruptive behaviors.	Small sample size. No blinding of evaluation. Short-term intervention.
http://dx.doi.org/10.1177/1362361307098516				

(Continued)

Table D.1. Evidence for Social–Emotional Development Interventions (*Cont.*)

Author/Year	Study Objectives	Level/Design/Participants	Intervention and Outcome Measures	Results	Study Limitations
Whalen et al. (2006)	To examine collateral changes in social initiations, positive affect, play, imitation, and language after participation of children with ASD in a joint attention training program	Level IV—Multiple baseline, single subject. *N* = 4 children with ASD and 6 peer models Mean age = 4 yr, 2 mo	*Intervention* The joint attention treatment used naturalistic behavior modification techniques that included discrete trial training and pivotal response training. The child was taught to respond to joint attention bids, then was taught to initiate joint attention bids. *Outcome Measures* • Unstructured Joint Attention Assessment, rated in 30 min of play • Structured Joint Attention Assessment, rated in Structured Play, Empathic Response, and Structured Play Assessment • Play and language were measured in 10-min probes.	The 4 participants showed increases in social initiations and positive affect at posttreatment; 3 improved in empathic response. All improved on the Structured Play Assessment. Imitation increased an average of 20%. No changes in the rate of functional or symbolic play. Improved joint attention may lead to increased attention to social stimuli.	Small sample size. No standardized assessments.

http://dx.doi.org/10.1007/s10803-006-0108-z

Interventions to Promote Peer-to-Peer Engagement

Betz et al. (2008)	To assess the use of a joint activity schedule to increase peer engagement for preschoolers with autism	Level IV—Multiple baseline, single subject. *Participants* *N* = 3 dyads, ages 4 and 5 yr, diagnosed with ASD	*Intervention* A joint photograph activity schedule was used from which the children chose the activity. Scripts were provided. The instructors guided the play. In baseline, the dyads were simply told to play. *Outcome Measures* The dyads were given interactive games. Independent observers scored at intervals whether the children were engaged, prompted, or unengaged.	The dyads' engagement was low during baseline and increased rapidly during teaching and persisted > 80% during the maintenance phases with no prompting. Playing with a designated peer according to a schedule reinforced event. Joint activity schedules may increase peer engagement and play among children with ASD.	Small sample size. No standardized assessments. No blinding of evaluation.

http://dx.doi.org/10.1901/jaba.2008.41-237

Reference	Purpose	Level/Design/Participants	Intervention/Outcome Measures	Results	Limitations
Guralnick et al. (2006)	To evaluate the effectiveness of a 2-yr comprehensive, developmentally oriented, highly individualized intervention	Level I—Randomized control trial. N = 90 (7 cohorts each yr) Intervention group, n = 46 with disabilities; Mean age = 64 mo; 74% male; IQ = 72 Control group, n = 44 with disabilities; Mean age = 64 months; IQ = 72	*Intervention* Used playgroups of children with and without disabilities; plan was individualized. Psychologists worked with family and school personnel. Comprehensive and highly individualized intervention included scripts for children and family consultation. Information about the control group was not provided. *Outcome Measures* • 30-min playgroup observations coded in 10-sec intervals • The Play Observation Scale was used to rate social participation. • The Individual Social Behavior Scale measured the targeted child's interactions with peers.	Both conditions improved over time with minimal differences by condition (intervention and control). Significant time effects included positive direct to peer, responsive to peer, and total positive behavior. When the groups were divided into high and low IQ, the low-IQ children in intervention improved more in positive interaction with peers. Although this intervention failed to show extensive effects on children's competence with peers, it may be preventive of social competence problems.	Intervention protocol not well specified.

http://dx.doi.org/10.1352/0895-8017(2006)111[336:PTPSDO]2.0.CO;2

Reference	Purpose	Level/Design/Participants	Intervention/Outcome Measures	Results	Limitations
Howard et al. (1996)	To investigate the effect of computer activities in the preschool classroom on children's play and social interaction	Level II—Two groups, nonrandomized. *Participants* N = 37 children with disabilities and Individual Family Service Plan or IEP goals Intervention group n = 22, age 18–36 mo Control group n = 15, age 36–60 mo	*Intervention* The children in the intervention group were taught to use computers during the school day. They were engaged in developmentally appropriate computer activities. The children in the control group were engaged in supervised play activities. *Outcome Measure* The Peer Play Scale was used to measure behavioral categories of social interaction. Ten 10-min observations were made during computer and noncomputer activities.	Toddlers and preschoolers demonstrated more active waiting, less solitary play, more turn taking, more attention to communication, and more positive affect during small-group computer activities than they did when engaged in small-group activities that did not involve the computer.	

(Continued)

Table D.1. Evidence for Social–Emotional Development Interventions (*Cont.*)

Author/Year	Study Objectives	Level/Design/Participants	Intervention and Outcome Measures	Results	Study Limitations
Kim et al. (2003)	To synthesize the findings of studies that examine the effects of toys and group composition on social behaviors of 3- to 5-yr-old children with disabilities	Level I—Systematic review of studies from 1975 to 1999. 13 studies met the criteria: 10 journal articles, 2 dissertations, 1 thesis, and 1 technical report. (One study was reported in two papers.)	*Intervention* Most studies compared the effects of isolate and social toys. Group composition studies examined mixed groups of children at different levels with groups in which the children were similar. *Outcome Measures* Social interaction, social behaviors, and cognitive play were measured in most studies.	Playing with social toys increased positive social outcomes more than playing with isolate toys for children with disabilities. Child-directed play was associated with more positive social behaviors than adult-directed play. Play groups including children with and without disabilities were associated with positive social outcomes for children with disabilities. Therapists should make social toys available in the classrooms and sessions should use small groups with children of different ability levels.	Combined disparate interventions. Most effects were low.
Tanta et al. (2005)	To examine the differences in initiation and response exhibited by preschool-age children with social-play delays when participating in dyads of differing developmental levels	Level IV—Single subject, alternating treatment. $N = 15$ $n = 5$ children at risk for developmental disabilities, 3 boys, 2 girls; age = 3.8–6.3 yr $n = 5$ peers developmentally 1 yr ahead $n = 5$ peers developmentally 1 yr behind	*Intervention* The at-risk children were engaged in free play with a peer who had higher level play skills or a peer with lower level play skills. All play dyads were in the same playroom. *Outcome Measures* The play was videotaped and coded for initiation and response at 30-sec intervals during the play session.	All children showed more initiation and response to initiation during play with higher level peers. For some children, the improvement was not immediate. Pairing a child with a developmentally higher peer can facilitate the emergence of social behaviors.	A more specified protocol may have resulted in larger effects. Small sample size.

http://dx.doi.org/10.1177/10538151030250304

http://dx.doi.org/10.5014/ajot.59.4.437

Social Skill Instruction

Crozier & Tincani (2007)	To examine the effect of a Social Story® intervention on children in an inclusive preschool and to assess the appropriateness of Social Stories with preschool children	Level IV—ABAB reversal design for 2 children and ABCACBC for 1. N = 3 boys with ASD; 2 were 3 yr, 9 mo, and 1 was 5 yr, 1 mo.	*Intervention* Target behaviors were identified that interfered with learning or socialization and were not being addressed with another intervention. Social Stories were written using the Social Story format. *Outcome Measures* Targeted behaviors were measured during 10-min sessions. Event recording was used.	Overall, inappropriate behaviors were reduced; appropriate behaviors and targeted skills increased. These increases were modest. Social Stories have modest positive effects on children with ASD.	Small sample size. Different behaviors were measured. Measured immediate but not retained behaviors.
http://dx.doi.org/10.1007/s10803-006-0315-7					
Hwang & Hughes (2000)	To systematically review studies of the effectiveness of social interactive training on early social communicative skills of children with an ASD	Level 1—Systematic review of 16 studies. N = 64 children with autism. 84% were boys. Age range = 2–12 yr; Mean age = 6.5 yr	*Intervention* Social interactive strategies used most often were (1) contingent imitation, (2) naturally occurring reinforcement, (3) *waiting for child's response, and (4)* environmental arrangement. *Outcome Measures* Most studies used direct observation of eye gaze; requesting action, object, or information; greetings; joint attention; expressing affection; imitative play; naming pictures; and verbal responding.	Time delay results in increases in verbal responses, greetings, and requesting skills. Environmental arrangement resulted in increases in requests, responses, and initiations and prolonged social interactions. Contingent imitation increased eye gaze, positive affect, and attending. Nine studies reported generalization of skills; five showed maintenance of positive findings. Combining these techniques can enhance children's engagement and social interaction skills.	Small number of studies included in the review.
http://dx.doi.org/10.1023/A:1005579317085					

(Continued)

Table D.1. Evidence for Social–Emotional Development Interventions (*Cont.*)

Author/Year	Study Objectives	Level/Design/Participants	Intervention and Outcome Measures	Results	Study Limitations
Kroeger et al. (2007)	To compare a direct teaching social skills group, using video modeling, to a play activity social skills group in children with ASD	Level II—Two group, non-randomized. N = 25 children with a diagnosis of ASD. Direct teaching group, n = 13, 9 boys, 4 girls; Mean age = 64 mo (SD = 12.3). Play group n = 12, 11 boys, 1 girl; Mean age = 61.4 mo (SD = 9.2)	*Intervention* Both groups participated in 15 hr/15 sessions. The direct teaching group received video modeling instruction, and members were prompted to generalize. The video modeling tapes were of 2 typical boys demonstrating motor imitation, ball play, taking turns, playing with partners, pretend. The play group had free play with peers. Behavioral techniques were used with both groups. *Outcome Measures* • Two trained graduate students coded the Social Interaction Observation Code measures of frequency, duration, and nature of videotaped social interactions. • Assessment of Basic Language and Learning Skills.	The direct teaching group made more gains in social skills than the play activities group and were higher in initiating, responding, and interacting behaviors. Factors contributing to the social gains seem to be the low student–facilitator ratio, the structured group format, and the well-trained facilitators. Video modeling provides a consistent way to teach a variety of skills.	Small sample size. No follow-up measures.
http://dx.doi.org/10.1007/s10803-006-0207-x					
Reichow & Volkmar (2010)	To examine the evidence of recently studied social skills interventions for preschool children with ASD	Level I—Systematic review. Of 66 studies that were reviewed, 35 (53%) studies included preschool children with ASD. N = 186 preschool children received intervention, 79% male	*Intervention* Interventions included parent training and peer training. Peers were taught to provide pivotal response treatment, visual supports, and prompting. Most interventions were administered by nonparental adults. ABA (prompting and reinforcement) was used most frequently. Therapy was provided in multiple sessions per week. Most interventions targeted social communication and social interaction. Setting included schools (19 studies), clinical settings, and homes. *Outcome Measures* Included standardized measures of social behavior (e.g., Vineland) and observational measures of behaviors.	Training peers to deliver treatment has strong support and is a recommended practice. Visual supports and visual modeling can be effective to enhance social understanding and to structure social interaction. Use of ABA techniques, including prompting and reinforcement, imitation and modeling, and self-monitoring, were effective practices.	Broad review of social interventions, most of which were used behavioral therapy. Limited application to occupational therapy.
http://dx.doi.org/10.1007/s10803-009-0842-0					

Vaughn et al. (2003)	To synthesize the findings for social skill interventions for 3- to 5-yr-old children with disabilities between 1975 and 1999	Level 1—Systematic review. 23 group design studies that met the following criteria: preschool children, identified disability, adequate design, and use of social skills interventions. $N = 699$ children with disabilities and 203 children without disabilities	*Intervention* Features of social skills interventions are prompting and rehearsal of target behaviors, play-related activities, free-play generalization, reinforcement of appropriate behaviors, modeling of specific social skills, storytelling, direct instruction of social skills, and imitation of appropriate behaviors. *Outcome Measures* The measures included observational tools that counted the frequencies that specific behaviors occurred.	Interventions with large effects and positive social outcomes included modeling, play-related activities, rehearsal or practice, and prompting. Reinforcement, free-play generalization, and direct instruction also were associated with large effect sizes. Improvements in social outcomes were achieved by social skills programs embedded into regular class programs, interventions that includes instruction and behavioral contingencies, and training parents or peers.	Broad review that includes studies of a variety of social skills interventions.

http://dx.doi.org/10.1177/07419325030240010

Note. ADHD = attention deficit hyperactivity disorder; ASD = autism spectrum disorder; IEP = individualized education program; *SD* = standard deviation.

This table is a product of AOTA's Evidence-Based Practice Project and the *American Journal of Occupational Therapy.* Copyright © 2013 by the American Occupational Therapy Association. It may be freely reproduced for personal use in clinical or educational settings as long as the source is cited. All other uses require written permission from the American Occupational Therapy Association. To apply, visit www.copyright.com.

Suggested citation: Case-Smith, J. (2013). Systematic review of interventions to promote social–emotional development in young children with or at risk disability (Suppl. Table 1). *American Journal of Occupational Therapy. 67.*

Table D.2. Evidence for Behavioral, Parent-Directed and Educational, and Physiological Interventions

Author/Year	Study Objectives	Level/Design/Participants	Intervention and Outcome Measures	Results	Study Limitations
Behavioral Interventions					
Benoit et al. (2000)	To assess the efficacy of a behavioral intervention in eliminating the need for enteral tube feeding in infants who no longer had a medical indication for this intervention but were resistant to oral feeding	Level I—Randomized control trial. $N = 64$ children age 4–36 mo who were tube fed and had resistance to feeding, behavioral, or nutritional interventions randomly allocated into 2 groups (32 per group, behavioral or nutritional intervention group)	*Intervention* Behavior (extinction/flooding) + nutritional intervention for 7 wk. *Outcome Measures* • Discontinuation of enterostomy tube feeding • Infant Feeding Behavior rater checklist, Infant Feeding Behavior parent checklist • Infants' weight and length.	At the 8-wk visit, 47% of patients in behavioral therapy were no longer dependent on tube feed. Participants in the behavioral group ingested a greater proportion of their daily energy requirements orally compared with the nutritional group at each of the following visits.	Limited generalizability; intervention would not be appropriate for children with uncoordinated swallowing. Not a blind study.
http://dx.doi.org/10.1067/mpd.2000.108397					
Byars et al. (2003)	To describe multicomponent feeding program outcomes with children who have Nissen fundoplication and feeding gastrostomy	Level III—One group, pre- and posttreatment, and follow-up comparison. $N = 9$ children with Nissen fundoplication and feeding gastrostomy	*Intervention* Short-term intensive biobehavioral treatment. *Outcome Measures* • Behavioral Pediatric Feeding Assessment Scale • Classification system for complex feeding disorder • Caloric intake (oral and G-tube), weight and height.	Successful in improving oral intake and weaning from gastrostomy tube feeding in children with Nissen fundoplication and feeding gastrostomy. The M percent ideal body weight for height was not compromised during intensive treatment.	Small sample size limits the generalizability. Lack of posttreatment measures of behavioral feeding resistance.
http://dx.doi.org/10.1097/00005176-200310000-00014					

Study	Study Objectives	Level/Design/Participants	Intervention and Outcome Measures	Results	Study Limitations
Greer et al. (2008) http://dx.doi.org/10.1093/jpepsy/jsm116	To investigate the effects of an intensive interdisciplinary feeding program on caregiver stress and child outcomes of children with feeding disorders across three categories	Level III—One-group pre- and postdischarge. N = 121 children in 3 categories (tube-dependent, liquid-dependent, or food-selective groups)	*Intervention* Inpatient (behavior therapy 3 hr/day and oral–motor therapy 1 hr/day, 7 days/wk) and day treatment program (behavior therapy 3 hr/day and oral–motor therapy 1 hr/day, 5 days/wk). Oral–motor therapy: Nutritive and nonnutritive oral–motor exercises. *Outcomes Measures* • Caregiver stress level • Child mealtime behaviors • Weight and calories.	Caregiver stress, child mealtime behaviors, weight, and caloric intake improved significantly after treatment in the intensive feeding program regardless of category placement.	Not randomized, discrepant sample size across the groups. No association between caregiver stress level and child program outcome. No long-term follow-up. Caregiver outcomes were measured at discharge. Decrease in caregiver stress could not be interpreted as a result of treatment effects.
Kerwin (1999)	To identify treatment studies for severe pediatric feeding problems	Level I—Systematic review. N = 79 peer-reviewed journal articles 1970–1997 (29 met the methodology criteria) Children ages birth to 18 yr with identified oral feeding problem. Studies investigating psychosocial or behavioral interventions, including medications, positioning, surgery, oral–motor treatment, oral–tactile stimulation.	*Interventions* Psychosocial or behavioral intervention. *Outcome Measures* Measure of eating or caloric ingestion.	Effective interventions for children with severe feeding problems are contingency management treatments that include positive reinforcement of appropriate feeding responses and ignoring or guiding inappropriate responses. Promising interventions include positive reinforcement for acceptance, not removing the spoon for refusal, and swallow-induction training.	The studies had various methodological limitations. Additional research is needed using either psychological placebo or established treatment as control conditions.

(Continued)

Table D.2. Evidence for Behavioral, Parent-Directed and Educational, and Physiological Interventions (*Cont.*)

Author/Year	Study Objectives	Level/Design/Participants	Intervention and Outcome Measures	Results	Study Limitations
Laud et al. (2009)	To evaluate treatment outcomes of an interdisciplinary feeding program	Level III—One group, nonrandomized. $N = 46$ children ages 36 to 145 mo (Mean age = 69 mo) with a diagnosis of autism spectrum disorder (ASD)	*Intervention* Inpatient (behavior therapy 3 hr/day and oral–motor therapy 1 hr/day × 7 days/wk) and day treatment program (behavior therapy 3 hr/day and oral–motor therapy 1 hr/day × 5 days/wk). Oral–motor therapy: nutritive and non-nutritive oral–motor exercises. *Outcome Measures* • *Participant feeding behaviors:* Acceptance, refusal behaviors, negative vocalizations, grams consumed. • *Caregiver assessment measures:* Children's Eating Behavior Inventory (CEBI), caregiver satisfaction scores. • *Follow-up:* Questionnaires on volume, variety, texture, mealtime refusal behavior and caregiver satisfaction.	Acceptance, refusal behaviors and grams consumed increased significantly; negative vocalizations significantly decreased from admission to discharge. A significant decrease in the total eating problem score (CEBI) from admission to discharge was found. At follow-up, the majority of the sample reported their children eating a greater variety of foods while engaging in less refusal.	Sample was not representative of most children with ASD. Efficacy of various treatment modalities in a less intensive outpatient setting for children with ASD should be evaluated. Follow-up data were assessed at only one point in time for each participant.

http://dx.doi.org/10.1177/01454450946729

Wilder et al. (2005)	To examine the use of noncontingent reinforcement to decrease self-injury and increase bite acceptance in a child who exhibited food refusal.	Level IV—Single-subject design. 40-mo-old girl diagnosed with autism, gastroesphageal reflux, and food allergies	*Intervention* Noncontingent reinforcement 2×/wk (10 min) for approximately 6 wk. *Outcome Measures* • Self-injury • Bite acceptance.	Results of the intervention showed a decrease in self-injury and an increase in bite acceptance.	Limited generalizability due to single-subject design.

http://dx.doi.org/10.1901/jaba.2005.132-04

Williams et al. (2007)	To describe a day treatment program that was developed as a more cost-effective alternative to inpatient treatment of severe feeding programs	Level III—One group. N = 46 children ages 16–133 mo (Mean age = 37 mo) with severe feeding problems with G-tubes	*Intervention* Intensive behavioral therapy in a day treatment program (contingency contacting, re-presentation, swallow induction, thermal stimulation, exit criterion, texture fading, response cost for refusal, differential reinforcement of other behavior, token economy, graduated guidance for self feeding, prompts for self feeding). *Outcome Measures* Oral intake and the need for tube feed at discharge, 12-, and 24-mo follow-up (*successful* = complete elimination of all tube feeding, *partially successful* = dependence on tube feedings for 50% or less of calories; *unsuccessful* = dependence on tube feedings for more than 50% of caloric needs)	67% of children were successfully weaned from their feeding tube during the course of treatment. 30% were partially successful, and 1 participant was not successful. At 1-yr follow up, 63% remained successful, 28% were partially successful and 9% unsuccessful. At 2-yr follow up, 74% were successful, 17% were partially successful, and 9% were unsuccessful.	Study was limited to examining the efficacy of intensive therapy and comparing the direct costs of feeding therapy and tube feeding. It did not compare the utilization of medical services for children who were tube fed but did not receive intensive therapy with that of children who receive intensive therapy. Did not measure psychosocial or other benefits of oral feeding for children or their families.

http://dx.doi.org/10.1007/s10882-007-9051-y

Parent-Directed and Educational Interventions

Black et al. (1995)	To evaluate the efficacy of a home-based intervention on the growth and development of children with nonorganic failure to thrive	Level I—Randomized control trial. N = 130 children Mean age = 12.7 ± 6.4 mo Intervention group n = 64 Control group n = 66	*Intervention* *Intervention group:* Clinic and home visit for 1 yr. Home visits were done by trained lay person. *Control group:* Clinic only. *Outcome Measures* • Growth • Language development • Parent–child behavior during feeding.	Children's weight for age, weight for height, and height for age improved significantly, regardless of intervention status. Children in the home intervention group had better receptive language over time than the clinic-only group. Significant improvements in children's interaction competence and parents' becoming more controlling during feeding regardless of intervention status, suggesting that intervention was not effective in altering maternal behavior	Intervention needs to combine with education and special service components.

(Continued)

Table D.2. Evidence for Behavioral, Parent-Directed and Educational, and Physiological Interventions *(Cont.)*

Author/Year	Study Objectives	Level/Design/Participants	Intervention and Outcome Measures	Results	Study Limitations
Chatoor et al. (1997)	Describe a developmental treatment model for infantile anorexia	Level III—*N* = 40 Intervention group *n* = 20 toddlers with infantile anorexia Control group *n* = 20 toddlers without infantile anorexia Followed 6 mo to 2 yr postintervention	*Intervention* 3 feeding sessions under supervision, follow-up phone call and visits. *Outcome Measures* • Feeding scale to assess mother–infant interaction • Weight and height • Interview with mothers.	17 mothers reported that they had relaxed over their children's food intake. Infants with anorexia increased their body weight 7% significantly.	Subjective assessment measures limited to only provide description. Limited generalizability.
http://dx.doi.org/10.1097/00001163-199704000-00004					
Fraser et al. (2004)	To evaluate the effectiveness of a single-session group, early intervention, multidisciplinary, education program designed to improve children's problem eating and mealtime behaviors	Level III—One-group, pretest–posttest. Convenience sample of 106 parents of children ages 2–10 yr who attended a food program conducted in community health venues	*Intervention* 2.5-hr education program that covers the main content areas of childhood nutrition and behavioral management strategies. *Outcome Measures* Children's Eating and Mealtime Behavior Inventory.	Significant improvement (with large effect size) in children's problem eating and mealtime behaviors after parent education program	13% of the studied sample were age 6 yr and older. Maturation effect. Lack of control group.
http://dx.doi.org/10.1177/0017896904630304					
Garcia Coll et al. (1996)	To assess the impact of an individualized behavioral feeding intervention with mothers on postnatal growth patterns in full-term infants (FT) and those who were intrauterine growth retarded (IUGR)	Level I—Randomized control trial. *N* = 61 infants Intervention group *n* = 27 IUGR Comparison group *n* = 34 FT Sample size was sufficient to detect medium to large effects with an alpha of 0.05.	*Intervention* Videotape of feeding interaction with feedback given to mother immediately following the feeding interaction in the context of viewing the selected video segments with the mother. *Outcome Measures* • Anthropometric measurements (weight, head circumference, length, skin fold thickness) • Formula intake.	Individualized behavioral feeding intervention can accelerate early growth in IUGR bottle-fed infants in the short term during the period of intervention (birth to 1 mo). On most parameters of physical growth, there is no lasting catch-up growth over the first 18 mo in IUGR infants.	Results cannot be generalized beyond bottle-fed infants. Unknown whether beneficial effects might have continued if the intervention had continued beyond the neonatal period.
http://dx.doi.org/10.1016/0378-3782(96)01748-3					

Pinelli et al. (2001)	To determine whether supplementary structured breastfeeding counseling (SSBC) for both parents compared with conventional hospital breastfeeding support (CHBS) improves the duration of breastfeeding in very low birthweight infants up to 1 yr old	Level I—Randomized control trial with longitudinal follow-up of infants at term and age 1, 3, 6, 12 mo. Parents of infants with birthweight < 1,500 g, who planned to breastfeed N = 128 Intervention group n = 64 SSBC couples Control group n = 64 CHBS couples	*Intervention* SSBC: Viewing a video on breastfeeding for preterm infants; individual counseling by the research lactation consultant; weekly personal contact in the hospital, and frequent postdischarge contact through the infants' first year. CHBS: Standard breastfeeding support from regular staff members during the period of hospitalization in the NICU. *Outcome Measures* Duration of breastfeeding.	No statistically significant difference in duration of breastfeeding between the two groups.	Participants in both re were highly motivated and committed to breastfeed.
Pridham et al. (2005) http://dx.doi.org/10.1002/nur.20073	To examine the effect of a method of supporting development on premature infant and maternal feeding competencies	Level I—Randomized control trial. 42 mother–infant pairs randomly assigned to either guided participation (GP) or standard care (SC) group	*Intervention* GP provided by a project nurse. Weekly home visits for the 1st month, then weekly, biweekly, or monthly for the 1st postterm yr. Phone calls between visits to answer questions. *Outcome Measures* • Child feeding skills for infant feeding skills • MPAB, MRNAB, IPAB, and IRNAB for maternal and infant feeding interaction competencies • Centers for Epidemiological Studies–Depression Scale for mothers' symptoms of depression.	GP significantly and positively contributed to MRNAB at 4 mo and to IRNAB at 1 and 8 mo. Negative effect of symptoms of depression on MRNAB at 8 mo.	Study's low power limits confidence in the adequacy of the study's assessment of GP effectiveness. Small sample size.

(Continued)

Table D.2. Evidence for Behavioral, Parent-Directed and Educational, and Physiological Interventions (*Cont.*)

Author/Year	Study Objectives	Level/Design/Participants	Intervention and Outcome Measures	Results	Study Limitations
Physiological Interventions					
Barlow et al. (2008)	To evaluate the effects of a new motorized pacifier to transition tube to oral feed	Level II—Two group, pre- and posttest. $N = 31$ tube-fed preterm infants Intervention group $n = 20$ Control group $n = 11$	*Intervention* *Intervention group:* 3-min epochs of patterned oral somatosensory stimulation during gavage feeds 3–4×/day. *Control group:* Regular pacifiers *Outcome Measures* Physical parameters of NNS and oral feed.	The patterned orocutaneous stimulus was highly effective in accelerating the development of NNS: minute rates for total oral compressions, bursts, NNS cycles, suck cycles per bursts. Greater success occurred in oral feeding than in the control group.	Small sample size. Did not investigate swallowing.
http://dx.doi.org/10.1038/jp.200857					
Bier et al. (1996)	To evaluate the effects of maternal–infant SSC vs standard contact (SC) on low-birthweight infants' physiological profile and duration of breastfeeding	Level I—Randomized control trial. Intervention study with cohort followed up for 6 mo after discharge $N = 50$ infants with birthweight <1,500 g randomized to 2 groups	*Intervention* *SSC group:* Infants were clothed in diaper and held upright between mother's breasts; both mother and infant were covered with a blanket. *SC group:* Infants were clothed, wrapped in blankets, and held cradled in mothers' arms. *Outcome Measures* • Physiological data • Duration of BF.	Infants in SSC group had higher oxygen saturation. 90% of mothers in SSC group continued BF for the duration of the infants' hospitalization, and 50% in the SSC group (vs 11% in the SC) continued breastfeeding through 1 mo after discharge.	Small sample size.
http://dx.doi.org/10.1001/archpedi.1996.02170370043006					
Boiron et al. (2007)	To compare the effects of oral stimulation with those of oral support on NNS and feeding parameters in preterm infants	Level I—Randomized control trial. $N = 43$ preterm infants <34 wk gestational age randomly allocated into one of the 3 experimental groups: stimulation + support ($n = 9$), stimulation ($n = 11$), and support ($n = 12$), or control group ($n = 11$)	*Interventions* 12 min of oral stimulation 1×/day 30 min before gavage for ≤14 consecutive days. Oral support was administered 2×/day for a maximum of 10 min. *Outcome Measure* NNS pressure using pressure transducer and sucking activity; time of transition, the quantity of milk ingested per day, and number of bottle feeds per day.	Oral stimulation delivered during gavage significantly enhanced the NNS parameters (NNS pressure and sucking activity). Oral support applied alone or combined with oral stimulation during the transition period improved NNS pressure and feeding parameters, and reduced the transition time.	Small sample size.
http://dx.doi.org/10.1111/j.1469-8749.2007.00439.x					

Study	Study Objectives	Level/Design/Participants	Intervention and Outcome Measures	Results	Study Limitations
Bragelien et al. (2007) http://dx.doi.org/10.1111/j.1469-8749.2007.00439.x	To study the effect of stimulation of sucking and swallowing on weaning from nasogastric (NG) feeding and length of hospital stay in premature infants	Level I—Randomized control trial with blinded evaluation. N = 36 preterm infants (<36 wk GA) on NG feedings Intervention and control group n = 18	*Intervention* Infants received stimulation based on Vojta's technique of initiating reflex activity of striate and smooth muscle for 15 min once a day. *Outcome Measures* • Infant age when NG feedings were discontinued • Infant age when discharged home.	There were no group differences in infants when NG feedings were discontinued or when infants were discharged home.	Small sample size resulting in limited statistical power. Treatment was given only once daily.
Einarsson-Backes et al. (1994) http://dx.doi.org/10.5014/ajot.48.6.490	To determine the effectiveness of oral support on feeding efficiency in preterm infants who were identified by the medical team as poor feeders	Level III—One group. *Participants* N = 13 premature infants between 34 and 40 wk GA who were selected from a group of infants at children's hospital and medical center in Seattle	*Intervention* Infants were fed twice, once with oral support and once without. The order of occurrence of these two conditions was randomly selected without replacement to ensure an equal number of both conditions. *Outcome Measure* Volume intake.	A statistically significant difference in volume intake occurred between the oral support condition and the no-oral-support condition.	The relatively short data collection periods (2 min) did not allow the examination of the effect of providing oral support over an entire feeding session. Small sample size. Limited number of data points.
Fucile et al. (2002) http://dx.doi.org/10.1067/mpd.2002.125731	To assess whether an oral stimulation program, before the introduction of oral feeding, enhances the oral feeding performance of preterm infants born between 26 and 29 wk GA	Level I—Two-group randomized control trial. N = 32 preterm infants receiving full-tube feeding	*Intervention* *Intervention group:* Oral stimulation program consisting of stimulation of the oral structure for 15 min (10 days, once a day). *Control group:* Received a sham stimulation program. *Outcome Measures* • Time to attainment of independent oral feeding • Number of days to reach 1 and 4 successful oral feedings per day • Overall intake rate of milk transfer • Length of hospital stay.	Independent oral feeding was attained significantly earlier in experimental group. Overall intake and rate of milk transfer were significantly greater over time in the experimental group than the control groups ($ps = .0002$ and $.046$, respectively). No significant difference in the length of hospital stay.	Although there are general guidelines for the management of oral feedings, there is no specific protocol for initiating and advancing oral feedings at the participating institution.

(Continued)

Table D.2. Evidence for Behavioral, Parent-Directed and Educational, and Physiological Interventions (*Cont.*)

Author/Year	Study Objectives	Level/Design/Participants	Intervention and Outcome Measures	Results	Study Limitations
Fucile et al. (2005)	To assess the effect of an oral stimulation program on the maturation of sucking skills of preterm infants	Level I—Two-group randomized control trial. *N* = 32 preterm infants at 28 wk GA	*Intervention* A daily 15-min oral stimulation program for 10 days before the start of oral feeding. *Outcome Measures* Oral feeding performance was assessed as a function of both clinical outcomes and sucking skills. Clinical outcomes included number of days to transition from tube to full oral feedings, overall intake, and rate of milk transfer. Sucking skills included the maturational level of the sucking pattern, sucking frequency, and amplitudes of suction and expression.	The experimental group achieved full oral feeding 7 days sooner than the control group and demonstrated greater overall intake, rate of milk transfer, and amplitude of the expression component of sucking. *Endurance,* defined as ability to sustain the same sucking stage, sucking burst duration, and suction and expression amplitudes throughout a feeding session was not significantly different between the two groups.	Small sample size. Development of additional interventions aimed at facilitating the development of other skills involved in oral feeding, such as enhancing the suction component, behavioral state, and respiratory control, may be of great importance in order to develop more efficacious feeding intervention strategies.
http://dx.doi.org/10.1017/S0012162205000290					
Gaebler & Hanzlik (1996)	To examine the effects of stroking and a perioral and intraoral prefeeding stimulation program on healthy, growing, preterm infants	Level II—Two-group, pretest–posttest Two groups of 9 randomly assigned, medically stable, preterm infants, born at 30–34 wk gestation, were selected. Intervention group *n* = 9 Control group *n* = 9	*Intervention* *Intervention group:* 5-min stroking protocol in addition to a perioral and intraoral stimulation program. *Control group:* 5-min stroking protocol before feeding. *Outcome Measures* • Nipple and partial nipple feeds • Revised Neonatal Oral Motor Assessment • Days of hospital stay • Nutritive intake.	Compared with control group, the experimental group had • Increased number of nipple feeds • Greater weight gain • Fewer days of hospital stay • Higher scores on the Revised Neonatal Oral Motor Assessment nutritive suck scale.	Findings cannot be generalized to preterm infant populations who are at greater medical risk.
http://dx.doi.org/10.5014/ajot.50.3.184					

Author (Year)	Study Objectives	Level/Design/Sample	Intervention and Outcome Measures	Results	Limitations
Gisel et al. (2003)	To examine whether pulmonary function would improve following 1 yr of intervention with optimal positioning for feeding, control of gastroesophageal reflux, and use of food textures to minimize aspiration from swallowing	Level IV—Descriptive studies that include analysis of outcomes (case series). N = 3 girls with cerebral palsy with severe motor impairment and spastic tetrapariesis ages 18–43 mo	*Intervention* Positioning the child for each meal in the position that was shown to minimize eliminate aspiration, as determined by videofluoroscopy (VF), for 12 mo. *Outcome Measures* • VF and 24-hr esophageal pH-monitoring • Pulmonary function.	2 of 3 girls showed improvement in respiratory functions.	Generalization is limited due to the sample size and study design.
Hake-Brooks & Anderson (2008) http://dx.doi.org/10.1891/0730-0832.27.3.151	To determine the effects of kangaroo care (KC) on breastfeeding status in mother–preterm infant dyads from postpartum through 18 mo	Level I—Randomized control trial. N = 66 mother–infant dyads Kangaroo care (KC) group n = 36 Control group n = 32	*Intervention* *Intervention group:* Mothers were encouraged to experience KC with their infants as soon as possible after birth and for as long as possible each time. *Control group:* Received standard nursery care. *Outcome Measures* Index of Breastfeeding Status at hospital discharge and at 1.5, 3, 6, 12, and 18 mo.	KC dyads breastfed significantly longer. More KC dyads breastfed at full exclusivity at discharge and at 1.5, 3, and 6 mo.	Breastfeeding duration and exclusivity during follow-up were based entirely on self-report by the mothers. Mothers from control group may not get same level of attention as KC group.
Jadcherla et al. (2009) http://dx.doi.org/10.11097/MPG.0b013e3181752ce7	To determine pharyngeoesophageal motility correlates in neonates with dysphagia and the impact of multidisciplinary feeding strategy	Level III—One group pre-post. N = 20 neonates with dysphagia with GA 31 ± 5 wk and evaluated at 49.9 ± 16.5 wk postmenstrual age.	*Intervention* Multidisciplinary feeding strategy includes postural adaptation, sensory modification, hunger manipulation, and operant conditioning methods. *Outcome Measures* Safe nipple feeding ability.	75% of infants (15/20) showed success feeding with occupational therapy intervention (NNS, positioning, oral feeding).	Potential confounder variables not controlled. Videofluoroscopic swallow study is limited because of the ethical issue.

(Continued)

Table D2. Evidence for Behavioral, Parent-Directed and Educational, and Physiological Interventions (*Cont.*)

Author/Year	Study Objectives	Level/Design/Participants	Intervention and Outcome Measures	Results	Study Limitations
Lamm et al. (2005)	To investigate and isolate the specific regional mechanical functions of the tongue during swallowing—"Tactile stimulation on the tongue"	Level III—One group. $N = 45$ infants and children with dysphagia and failure to thrive ages 4 mo to 9.2 yr.	*Intervention* • A tactile stimulus to the posterior tongue. • Sequential tactile stimuli to varied locations on the lingual surface. *Outcome Measures* • Frequency and rate per minute (rpm) of swallow responses • *Oral consumption*, defined as rate per minute (rpm) cc, *M* bolus size consumed, and variety of oral consumption.	Tactile stimulation to the posterior tongue can induce swallow.	Additional research is needed to facilitate parental compliance and decrease drift from training procedures in the home environment, because parent training is a critical component for maintaining the patients' oral feeding gains in generalized settings. A biopsychosocial evaluation should be conducted to evaluate the patient and parents to determine social and psychological stresses contributing to dysphagia.

http://dx.doi.org/10.1007/s00455-005-0060-7

Author/Year	Study Objectives	Level/Design/Participants	Intervention and Outcome Measures	Results	Study Limitations
Larnert & Ekberg (1995)	To investigate whether trunk and neck positioning influenced oral and pharyngeal swallow	Level IV—Single-subject design. $N =$ convenience sample of 5 children with cerebral palsy aged 3–10 yr with history of swallowing problems	*Intervention* Two different sitting positions: upright and 30º backward with neck flexed. *Outcome Measures* Elements observed in Videoradiographic study: oral leak, pharyngeal swallow, aspiration.	In the reclined position with the neck flexed, aspiration decreased in all 5 children, oral leak diminished in 2 children, and retention improved in 1 child.	Small sample size. Lack of objective outcome measures (e.g., the amount of bolus was not assessed).

http://dx.doi.org/10.1111/j.1651-2227.1995.tb13730.x

Author/Year	Study Objectives	Level/Design/Participants	Intervention and Outcome Measures	Results	Study Limitations
Moore et al. (2009)	To assess the effects of early SSC on breastfeeding, behavior, and physiological adaptation in healthy mother–newborn dyads	Level I—Systematic review. $N = 30$ quasirandomized clinical trials involving 1,925 participants	Interventions include birth SSC, very early SSC, early SSC *Outcome Measures* Breastfeeding status and duration, success of the first breastfeeding, changes in infant physiological parameters during and after SSC, infant stabilization, hospital length of stay, behavior changes, and maternal bonding attachment behaviors.	A statistically significant positive effect on the success of the first breastfeeding, breastfeeding status Day 3 postbirth, breastfeeding 1 to 4 mo postbirth, breastfeeding duration was found for mothers and their healthy full-term or late preterm newborn infants (34–37 wk GA) who have early SSC starting less than 24 hr after birth.	Limitations in design, outcome variability, and long-term outcomes.

Munakata et al. (2008)	To assess whether black pepper oil (BPO) stimulation facilitates oral intake in pediatric patients receiving long-term enteral nutrition	Level III—Single-group design. N = 10 patients ages 19–97 mo requiring enteral nutrition.	*Intervention* The effects of scenting with BPO for 1 min immediately before every meal were evaluated. *Outcome Measures* Oral intake and some clinic observation (drooling, swallowing movements).	Eight patients completed 3-mo BPO intervention; 5 showed a distinct increase in oral intake. The increase was accompanied by desirable effects, such as facilitated appetite, reduced drooling, and distinct swallowing movements. BPO intervention was not effective in the other 3 patients.	Low evidence level. Case study.
Pinelli & Symington (2005)	To determine whether NNS in preterm infants influences physiologic stability and nutrition	Level I—Systematic review. N = 21 studies, 15 of which were randomized control trials All studies used experimental or quasi-experimental designs in which NNS in preterm infants was compared with no provision of NNS.	*Intervention* NNS *Outcome Measures* Weight gain, energy intake, heart rate, oxygen saturation, length of stay, intestinal transit time, age at full oral feed, other clinical outcomes.	NNS was found to decrease the length of hospital stay in preterm infants significantly. The review did not reveal a consistent benefit of NNS with respect to other major clinical variables (weight gain, energy intake, heart rate, oxygen saturation, intestinal transit time, age at full oral feeds, behavioral state). The review identified other positive clinical outcomes of NNS: transition from tube to bottle feeds and better bottle-feeding performance. No negative outcomes were reported in any of the studies.	8 of 15 studies were cross-over design. The washout time for NNS is unknown. Only 6 of 15 studies were clearly blinded.

http://dx.doi.org/10.1002/14651858.CD001071

(Continued)

Table D.2. Evidence for Behavioral, Parent-Directed and Educational, and Physiological Interventions (Cont.)

Author/Year	Study Objectives	Level/Design/Participants	Intervention and Outcome Measures	Results	Study Limitations
Poore et al. (2008)	To determine whether Ntrainer-patterned oro-cutaneous therapy affects preterm infants' NNS and/or oral feeding success	Level II—Two-group, pretest-posttest. *N* = 31 preterm infants with minimal NNS output and delayed transition to oral feeds at 34 wk. Intervention group *n* = 21. Control group *n* = 10	*Intervention* NTrainer treatment provided to 21 infants 4× per day during scheduled gavage feeds. *Outcome Measures* NNS nipple compression waveforms and percentage of oral feeding.	Treated infants manifest a disproportionate increase in suck pattern stability and percent oral feeding beyond that attributed to maturational effects alone.	Small sample size. This study was conducted on healthy preterm infants. The results cannot be generalized to preterm infants with greater medical complications (i.e., IVH 3–4).

http://dx.doi.org/10.1111/j.1651-2227.2008.00825.x

Reid (2004)	To identify feeding interventions recommended for infants with cleft conditions	Level I—Systematic review. *N* = 55 Level I–IV articles published 1955–2002	*Interventions* Early feeding and nutrition education as well as assisted feeding methods for infants with isolated cleft conditions. *Outcome Measures* Feeding method, mothers' reported ease and pleasure of feeding and estimate of infant contentment. Mean energy, protein intakes, growth, time to feed, weight gain, failure to thrive.	There are currently no completed systematic reviews relevant to this body of literature (Level I evidence). Two well-designed RCTs (Level I evidence) were found. These were considered to provide the strongest evidence for feeding intervention techniques. These articles described a combination of interventions, including early feeding and nutrition education as well as assisted feeding methods for infants with isolated cleft conditions. Three examples of Level III evidence were also found. Fifty (91%) of 55 articles reviewed were non–data-driven reports of expert opinion (Level IV).	High proportion of studies are Level V, expert opinion (50/55).

http://dx.doi.org/10.1597/02-148.1

Rocha et al. (2007)	To assess whether sensory–motor stimulation and NNS gavage feeding enhances the oral feeding performance of preterm infants born 26–32 wk GA	Level 1—Double-blind, two-group. Randomized control trial. *N* = 98 very low birth-weight infants randomized into a experimental and control group	*Intervention* *Experimental group:* Sensory–motor oral stimulation and NNS. *Control group:* Sham stimulation program. *Outcome Measure* Length of hospital stay.	Independent oral feeding was attained significantly earlier in the experimental group than the control group. There was significant difference in length of hospital stay between the two groups.	Study did not describe "sham stimulation" for the control group. Study was not designed to compare whether this intervention was of more benefit than NNS alone. Further studies are needed to verify this question.
http://dx.doi.org/10.1016/j.earlhumdev.2006.08.003					
Simpson et al. (2002)	To determine whether transition from tube to all-oral feeding can be accelerated by the early introduction of oral feeding in preterm infants	Level 1—Randomized control trial. *N* = 29 infants (<30 wk GA) randomly assigned to intervention and control groups	*Intervention* Oral feeding initiated 48 hr after full tube feed; the feeding progression followed a structured protocol. *Outcome Measures* • Milk transfer rate • Transition time from full tube feeding to all-oral feeding.	Infants in the experimental group were introduced to oral feeding significantly earlier than the control group and attained all-oral feeding significantly earlier as well.	Small sample size.
http://dx.doi.org/10.1542/peds.110.3.517					

(Continued)

Table D.2. Evidence for Behavioral, Parent-Directed and Educational, and Physiological Interventions (*Cont.*)

Author/Year	Study Objectives	Level/Design/Participants	Intervention and Outcome Measures	Results	Study Limitations
White-Traut et al. (2002)	To determine whether an auditory, tactile, visual, and vestibular intervention increases the proportion of alert behavioral states, thereby improving their feeding progression	Level I—Randomized control trial. *N* = 37 preterm infants (12 infants born at 23–26 wk gestation with normal head ultrasounds and 25 CNS-injured infants born at 23–31 wk) Intervention group *n* = 21 (7 males, 14 females) Control group *n* = 16 (11 males, 5 females) Infants were randomly assigned to groups at 32 wk postconceptional age.	*Intervention* *Intervention group:* Standard of nursing care, plus an auditory, tactile, visual, and vestibular intervention (ATVV). ATVV intervention provides infant-directed talk via a soothing female voice (auditory stimulation) as the researcher massages the infant for 10 min (tactile stimulation), followed by 5 min horizontal rocking (vestibular stimulation). Throughout the 15-min period, the researcher attempts to engage in eye contact with the infant (visual stimulation). *Control group:* Standard of nursing care, which included a stress reduction program *Outcome Measures* • Behavioral state • Feeding progression (proportion of nipple feeding to total intake).	Study group demonstrated increased alertness during the first 5 min of intervention, significantly correlated to length of stay. The proportion of nipple intake increased significantly faster for study group.	Small sample size. High rate of attrition due to hospital discharge. A significantly greater proportion of females were randomized to the study group.

http://dx.doi.org/10.1017/S0012162201001736

Note. *Behavioral Interventions* are defined as treatment strategies that are based on operant learning principles. Seven studies were categorized as research on behavioral interventions, including 2 Level I, 4 Level III, and 1 Level IV articles. Intervention strategies developed that address children's feeding problems by providing primary caregivers with information and recommendations regarding how to facilitate appropriate feeding behaviors were reviewed in the category of parent-directed and educational interventions. Six studies were categorized as research on parent-directed or educational interventions, including 4 Level I studies and 2 Level III studies. Interventions that concentrated on improving children's biological development, including physical and sensory functions to support infant feeding, were categorized as physiological interventions. Twenty-one studies were categorized as research on physiological interventions, including 12 Level I studies, 3 Level II studies, 4 Level III studies, and 2 Level IV studies. GA = gestational age; IPAB = infant positive affect and behavior; IRNAB = infant regulation of negative affect and behavior; MPAB = maternal positive affect and behavior; MRNAB = maternal regulation of negative affect and behavior; NNS = non-nutritive sucking; SSC = skin-to-skin contact.

This table is a product of AOTA's Evidence-Based Practice Project and the *American Journal of Occupational Therapy.* Copyright © 2013 by the American Occupational Therapy Association. It may be freely reproduced for personal use in clinical or educational settings as long as the source is cited. All other uses require written permission from the American Occupational Therapy Association. To apply, visit www.copyright.com.

Suggested citation: Howe, T.-H., & Wang, T.-N. (2013). Systematic review of interventions used in or relevant to occupational therapy for children with feeding difficulties ages birth–5 years (Suppl. Table 1). *American Journal of Occupational Therapy, 67.*

Table D.3. Evidence for Interventions Used in Occupational Therapy to Promote Motor Performance

Author/Year	Study Objectives	Level/Design/Participants	Intervention and Outcome Measures	Results	Study Limitations
Developmental or Caregiver-Focused Interventions for Children With Motor Delays					
Blauw-Hospers & Hadders-Algra (2005) http://dx.doi.org/10.1017/S0012162205000824	To examine the elements of early intervention that contribute to motor development and to determine whether there is a critical age at which the intervention should begin	Level 1—Systematic review. $N = 34$; 17 studies were completed in neonatal intensive care units and 17 were post-NICU studies. Infants with high biological risk for or with developmental disabilities; age range = 0–18 mo corrected age	*Intervention* Categorized as sensory stimulation, motor intervention strategies, or parent–infant interaction strategies (e.g., NDT, NIDCAP). *Outcome Measures* Neuromotor or developmental.	This study moves forward from previous studies resulting in inconclusive results. Positive results were demonstrated in 13 of 34 studies.	The number of participants and level of rigor for each study varied.
Chiarello & Palisano (1998)	To examine the effectiveness of motor play treatments in the home with the mother and child vs. conventional therapy using interactive play treatments	Level 1—Randomized control trial. $N = 38$ mothers and their children. Children's age range = 6–34 mo	*Intervention* 5-wk parent education and behavioral intervention therapy treatments. *Outcome Measures* Child's behavior, child's mobility, mother's interaction, and the child and mother's summary measure.	The experimental group showed improvements in correctly holding and positioning their child and controlling their child's behavior. The control group promoted motor skills during interactive play.	Limited generalizability. Results for the mothers' behaviors were inconsistent. Participants received interventions to promote motor skills before the study.
Lekskulchai & Cole (2001)	To evaluate the effect of a motor developmental program in improving motor performance in Thai infants born preterm	Level 1—Randomized control trial. $N = 84$ preterm infants; gestational age of < 37 wk; randomly assigned to either a control or an intervention group Comparative group $n = 27$ infants who scored ≥ 67 on the Test of Infant Motor Performance (TIMP) at 40 wk gestational age	*Intervention* Home-based program implemented by caregivers after a demonstration and practice session were provided. Interventions were provided at 1, 2, and 3 mo adjusted age. *Outcome Measure* TIMP assessed motor performance monthly.	Infants who received the motor developmental program showed significantly greater improvements in motor performance during the study period than the infants in the control groups. At 4 mo adjusted age, the motor performance of the infants in the intervention group did not differ significantly from the not-at-risk preterm infants (the comparative group).	The effectiveness of the program relied heavily on the caregivers' understanding and cooperation with the protocol.

(Continued)

Table D.3. Evidence for Interventions Used in Occupational Therapy to Promote Motor Performance (*Cont.*)

Author/Year	Study Objectives	Level/Design/Participants	Intervention and Outcome Measures	Results	Study Limitations
McManus & Kotelchuck (2007)	To evaluate the effectiveness of aquatic therapy supplementing an early intervention program with children diagnosed with neuromuscular and developmental delays and disabilities, specifically focusing on functional mobility	Level II—Cohort nonrandomized controlled trial. $N = 37$ children (6–30 mo) with neuromuscular and developmental delays and disabilities Intervention group $n = 15$ Control group $n = 22$	*Intervention* Aquatic therapy intervention was provided 1x/wk for 30 min in addition to 60-min home session by both an occupational therapist and a physical therapist to 2 children simultaneously to treat individually and allow peer socialization. Control group received a 60-min home session each wk. *Outcome Measures* Gross Motor Subscale of the Mullen Scales of Early Learning.	Children who received aquatic therapy in conjunction with home-based early intervention services showed greater gains in functional mobility than the children receiving only home-based intervention. The results were not statistically significant.	Small sample size. The nature of the Gross Motor Subscale of the Mullen Scales of Early Learning may limit results. The participants in the study did not allow for generalizability. Study lacked randomization.
http://dx.doi.org/10.1097/PEP.0b013e3181575190					
Orton et al. (2009)	To examine the effects of early developmental intervention after discharge from the hospital on motor and cognitive development in preterm infants	Level I—Systematic review. Participants of each included study were infants born at < 37 wk gestational age with no major congenital abnormalities. 17 studies examined outcomes in infancy and school-age; 11 were included in the meta-analysis.	*Intervention* Infant interventions to improve cognitive or motor outcomes, performed in the hospital, home, or community center. Goals included parent–infant relationships and/or infant development. *Outcome Measures* Outcomes assessed using motor or cognitive measures.	Early developmental interventions improved cognitive outcomes at infants' age and at preschool age. The results were not sustained at school age. Early intervention had little effect on motor outcomes. Benefits of developmental intervention may be restricted to short-term gains in cognitive outcomes.	Outcomes compiled were diverse; of 17 studies, only 9 had data analysis sufficient to include in the meta-analysis.
http://dx.doi.org/10.1111/j.1469-8749.2009.03414.x					
Interventions for Children With CP					
Sakzewski et al. (2009)	To determine the effectiveness of upper-limb interventions used with children diagnosed with congenital hemiplegia on activity and participation outcomes	Level I—Meta-analysis. $N = 13$ RCTs and 7 systematic reviews of children diagnosed with congenital hemiplegia ages 18 mo–16 yr.	*Intervention* Studies were categorized into four groups: (1) NDT, (2) CIMT and forced-use therapy, (3) hand–arm bimanual intensive training (HABIT), and (4) intramuscular botulinum toxin A (BoNT–A) injections. *Outcome Measures* Standardized and nonstandardized assessments grouped as upper-limb function, self-care, and individualized outcomes.	No clear strength of any 1 study over the other is stated. BoNT–A in conjunction with additional upper-limb training is growing in evidence of effectiveness. NDT has limited evidence. Both CIMT and HABIT are emerging interventions with positive evidence to support their effectiveness.	Small sample size. The treatment protocols, intensity, and duration varied among studies. Outcome measures varied among studies, and not all measures reported reliability and validity.
http://dx.doi.org/10.1542/peds.2008-3335					

Neurodevelopmental Motor Treatment

Author/Year	Study Objectives	Level/Design/Participants	Intervention and Outcome Measures	Results	Study Limitations
Arndt et al. (2008)	To evaluate the efficiency of an NDT-based sequenced trunk coactivation protocol for change in gross motor function in infants with posture and movement dysfunction	Level II—Repeated-measures randomized block design. NDT-based coactivation trunk protocol (STA), $n = 5$ children ages 4–12 mo. Parent–infant play protocol (PIP), $n = 5$	*Intervention* STA group intervention emphasized transitional activities. PIP group intervention emphasized parent–infant interaction, and enriched direct play. All participants also received early intervention services per their Individual Family Service Plan. *Outcome Measures* GMFM	The STA protocol group made significantly greater gains in gross motor function than the PIP protocol group. The STA protocol group maintained motor gains at the 3-wk follow-up session.	Small sample size. Throughout the duration of the study, the infants in both groups received ongoing early intervention therapeutic services.
http://dx.doi.org/10.1097.PEP/0b013e31815e8595					
Brown & Burns (2001)	To determine whether NDT for pediatric patients with neurological dysfunction is effective in modifying sensory input, inhibiting primitive reflexes, or inhibiting abnormal movements	Level I—Systematic review. $N = 17$ articles Participants were birth–14 yr, had a diagnosis of neurological dysfunction, and were involved in a NDT program. Six articles had sample sizes of ≥ 50, and 11 used control groups.	*Intervention* All articles incorporated NDT as the intervention to be evaluated. Of the interventions, 12 included a home program in addition to individual therapy; 3 included casting. *Outcome Measures* Outcomes for each article varied greatly, with numerous assessments being used. Examples include Peabody Developmental Motor Scale, goniometry, Bayley Scales of Infant and Toddler Development, Modified Ashworth Scale.	Six of the articles reported statistically significant results from the NDT treatment 9 reported no benefit. In 2 studies, the findings were equivocal. The evidence as to whether NDT is an effective treatment for children with neurological dysfunction was determined to be inconsistent; therefore NDT remains an experimental intervention.	Lack of an extensive literature search and studies with rigorous study designs.
Girolami & Campbell (1994)	To determine improvements of motor control in infants born prematurely and at risk for developmental delays through the use of an NDT protocol	Level I—Randomized control trial. *Participants* $N = 19$ infants born prematurely Control group $n = 8$	*Intervention* The full-term control group received no intervention services. The intervention group received treatment for 7–17 days focusing on facilitation of movement and strength for posture. The second preterm intervention group received nonspecific handling treatments for 7–17 days. *Outcome Measures* • Neonatal Behavioral Assessment Scale (NBAS) • Supplemental Motor Test (SMT).	Significant differences were found using the SMT in specific areas such as spontaneous movement and initiation of movement toward objects. No significant differences were found using the NBAS between the two preterm groups.	Small sample size. Infants were not tested again for long-term benefits.

(Continued)

Table D.3. Evidence for Interventions Used in Occupational Therapy to Promote Motor Performance (*Cont.*)

Author/Year	Study Objectives	Level/Design/Participants	Intervention and Outcome Measures	Results	Study Limitations
Law et al. (1991)	To determine the effects that intensive NDT and casting (separately and simultaneously) have on hand function, upper-extremity quality of movement, and range of motion when used with children diagnosed with spastic CP	Level I—Randomized control trial, two-by-two factorial design. $N = 72$ children ages 18 mo–8 yr *Groups:* Intensive NDT plus cast, $n = 19$; regular NDT plus cast, $n = 17$; intensive NDT, $n = 18$; regular NDT, $n = 18$.	*Intervention* Occupational therapists provided various interventions among groups. The intensive group received NDT twice weekly for 45 min, with a 30-min daily home program. These children also wore a cast on their more involved arm for at least 4 hr/day. The regular NDT group received in-clinic services between 1x/wk and 1x/mo, with a home program for 15 min 3x/wk. *Outcome Measures* • PFMS • QUEST.	The PFMS did not demonstrate significant differences at any time among any of the treatment groups. Quality of movement (QUEST) results (6 mo) showed children in the inhibitive casting groups obtained significantly higher results, and then they decreased (9 mo). No statistical significance was found. Children with casted arm had a significant increase in wrist extension.	Sample size limited the study's power. The attendance rate among the groups may have influenced the results.

http://dx.doi.org/10.1111/j.1469-8749.1191.tb14897.x

Law et al. (1997)	To determine the effectiveness of NDT and casting in improving hand function, quality of upper-extremity movement, and range of motion in children with CP	Level II—Cohort study. $N = 50$ children 18 mo–4 yr (mean age = 32.92 mo) with CP (22 diplegia, 19 hemiplegia, 9 quadriplegia) $N = 42$ participants in therapy before beginning the study NDT plus casting group, $n = 26$ Regular OT group, $n = 24$	*Intervention* Focused on changing impairments and improving upper-extremity quality of movement. 45 min OT twice, 30-min home program. *Control group:* The OT program focused on task analysis and change in functional skills and met 45 min 1x/wk Both conditions were administered by trained occupational therapist. Duration was 12 months. *Outcome Measures* • COPM • QUEST • PFMS.	No significant results were found for hand function, quality of upper-extremity movement, or parents' perception of hand function between the 2 groups.	Small sample size. 42 participants were receiving therapy before the intervention.

http://dx.doi.org/10.1111/j.1469-8749.1997.tb07360.x

Study	Level/Design	Intervention and Outcome Measures	Results	Limitations
Mayo (1991)	Level I—Randomized control trial. N = 29 Intensive NDT group, n = 17, Mean age = 11.4 mo Basic NDT group, n = 12, Mean age = 9.9 mo	To compare the changes in development over a 6-mo period of weekly (intensive) and monthly (basic) NDT on the motor development of young children with suspected CP *Intervention* Both regimes lasted 6 mo. The basic regime consisted of monthly hospital visits at which the parents received instructions for carrying out a home program. The intensive regime occurred weekly, allowing the therapist to implement special maneuvers to meet specific therapeutic goals. *Outcome Measures* • Reflex activity • Postural reactions • Gross motor ability • Fine motor skills • Bayley Scales of Infant and Toddler Development Mental scale • Abnormal movement scale • ADLs.	The average proportional change in aggregate motor development for the infants in the intensive group was significantly better than for the infants in the basic regime, after adjusting for the child's age, whether the child was born at term, and mother's education.	Findings were limited by small sample size. The groups did not have similar demographics. Only two of the seven instruments used were known to be valid and reliable. Compliance was not measured. Some infants were included whose final diagnosis was not CP.

http://dx.doi.org/10.1097/00002060-199110000-00006

Constraint-Induced Movement Therapy for Children With Unilateral CP

Study	Level/Design	Intervention and Outcome Measures	Results	Limitations
Aarts et al. (2010)	Level I—Randomized control trial. N = 50 children with diagnosis of CP with unilateral or severely asymmetric bilateral spastic movement impairment; ages = 2.5–8 yr; MACS scores I, II, or III Intervention (mCIMT) group n = 28 Control group n = 22	To investigate whether 6 wk of mCIMT followed by 2 wk of bimanual training in children with unilateral spastic CP improves spontaneous use of the affected limb in quantitative and qualitative measures when compared with usual care *Intervention* Children in the intervention group received mCIMT for 3 3-hr sessions/wk for 6 wk, followed by 2 wk task-specific training in goal-directed bimanual play and self-care activities. Children in the control group received usual care, which included 1.5 hr of general PT or OT and encouragement to use affected limb. *Outcome Measures* Primary: • Assisting Hand Assessment • ABILHAND–Kids. Secondary: • Melbourne Assessment of Unilateral Upper Limb Function • COPM • Goal Attainment Scaling.	All primary and secondary outcome measures, except the Melbourne Assessment, demonstrated significant improvements for the mCIMT–BiT group when compared with controls.	Most of the children had good arm–hand capacity (73.6% had MACS scores of I or II; decreases ability to generalize results). Follow-up was only 8 wk posttreatment, which makes judging long-term effects difficult in this study.

http://dx.doi.org/10.1177/1545968309359767

(Continued)

Table D.3. Evidence for Interventions Used in Occupational Therapy to Promote Motor Performance (*Cont.*)

Author/Year	Study Objectives	Level/Design/Participants	Intervention and Outcome Measures	Results	Study Limitations
Aarts et al. (2011) http://dx.doi.org/10.1016/j.ridd.2010.10.008	To investigate how improvements in spontaneous use of the affected limb during play and self-care activities were established as a result of 8 wk mCIMT and BiT	Level I—Randomized control trial. $N = 50$ children with diagnosis of CP with unilateral or severely asymmetric bilateral spastic movement impairment; ages = 2.5–8 yr; MACS scores I, II, or III Intervention (mCIMT) group, $n = 28$ Control group $n = 22$	*Intervention* Children in the intervention group received mCIMT for 3 3-hr sessions/wk for 6 wk, followed by 2 wk task-specific training in goal-directed bimanual play and self-care activities. Children in the control group received usual care, which included 1.5 hr of general PT or OT and encouragement to use affected limb. *Outcome Measures* Using video, developmental disregard and upper-limb capacity and performance were assessed. Goniometer measurements of PROM and AROM of the affected wrist and elbow, which were measured.	Children in the mCIMT–BiT group improved the spontaneous use of the upper limb during play and self-care activities more than those in the usual-care group. The improvements reflect increased use of existing motor functions rather than true restoration of muscle strength or motor selectivity. Results include improved quality and increased frequency of use, but not increased endurance or improved automaticity.	Only AROM and PROM at wrist and elbow of affected limb were measured as important underlying motor functions. Motor planning (cognition) was not specifically assessed in this study. Possible Type II error related to effects on developmental disregard.
DeLuca et al. (2006) http://dx.doi.org/10.1177/0883073806021011040i	To test the efficacy of pediatric CI therapy by means of a randomized controlled crossover trial (using the control group from Taub et al., 2004, study)	Level I—Randomized controlled cross-over trial. Intervention group, $n = 7$, ages 14–86 mo with a diagnosis of CP with asymmetric involvement of the upper extremity	*Intervention* All children from the control group in the Taub et al. (2004) study were crossed over into the CI therapy group. Children's less-impaired upper extremities were fully casted. Using shaping, an OT or PT provided 6 hr of therapy per day for 21 consecutive days. *Outcome Measures* The outcomes of the posttreatment from Phase I (Taub et al. study) served as the baseline for Phase 2. Children in the cross-over condition participated in 2 additional posttreatment assessments after CI therapy. • QUEST • PMAL • EBS.	This study's data demonstrated a similar pattern of results on frequency and quality of use on the PMAL (compared with the Taub et al. treatment group) and increased emergence of behaviors on the EBS. Control groups had no significant change.	Cross-over design has risks of carry over, learning effects, or both, which may affect results.

Taub et al. (2004)	To determine whether full application of both components of CI therapy protocol (extensive, intensive training of the more-affected arm and restraint of less-affected arm) would produce improvements in motor function in young children with CP	Level 1—Randomized control trial. Intervention, *n* = 8 children ages 7–85 mo (Mean age = 39.0 mo) Control group, *n* = 8 children ages 14–96 mo (Mean age = 43.4 mo)	*Intervention* Children in CIMT had their less-impaired upper extremity casted from upper arm to fingertips using a bivalve cast. The CIMT consisted of therapists' "shaping" new motor performance in 6 hr of therapy per day for 21 consecutive days. The children in the control group received PT, OT, or both for a mean of 2.2 hr/wk. *Outcome Measures* Immediately after intervention and 3 mo and 6 mo postintervention: • EBS • PMAL • TAUT • Developmental Activities Screening Inventory–II.	Children who participated in CIMT improved more in motor function than controls. Improvements include new motor patterns and classes of functional activity on EBS, improved amount and quality of use on the PMAL, and increased use of impaired upper extremity on TAUT.	This study had a small sample size. Positive findings may relate to time spent in treatment (intensity and frequency) vs. the constraint and intervention protocol. The dosage of intervention seemed high.

http://dx.doi.org/10.1542/peds.113.2.305

Willis et al. (2002)	To determine whether restraint of the unimpaired arm would improve function of the impaired arm in children with chronic (> 1 yr) hemiparesis	Level 1—Randomized control trial. Ages 1–8 yr Intervention group *n* = 7 Control group *n* = 10	*Intervention* The intervention group received a plaster cast on their unimpaired arm for 1 mo. The control group did not. Both groups continued their routine visits to occupational and PT; no effort was made to change their routines. *Outcome Measures* • PDMS at entry, 1 mo (when casts initially removed), 6 mo, and 7 mo after entry. • Parental report.	Children's use of their hemiparetic upper extremity improved after 1 mo of forced use in the intervention group of children.	Some participants received additional occupational and PT sessions; however, the researchers suggested that this did not improve results.

http://dx.doi.org/10.1542/peds.110.1.94

(Continued)

Table D.3. Evidence for Interventions Used in Occupational Therapy to Promote Motor Performance (*Cont.*)

Author/Year	Study Objectives	Level/Design/Participants	Intervention and Outcome Measures	Results	Study Limitations
Conductive Education					
Catanese et al. (1995)	To evaluate the effectiveness of a CE-based program for children with CP	Level II—Cohort study, nonrandomized. *N* = 34 children ages 4–7 yr with a diagnosis of CP and intellectual disability CE group *n* = 17 Control group *n* = 17	*Intervention* CE group: Combined education and therapy. Control group: Individual physiotherapy specifics of both groups not reported. Frequency and duration not stated *Outcome Measures* • VAB • Questionnaire on Resources and Stress, Short Form.	Both groups improved on gross motor function cognitive ability, receptive and expressive language, and grooming, with the CE group improving more than the control group on gross motor function. Caregivers reported improvements over time for both groups, with the CE group improving more on toileting and the control group improving more on social interaction and play.	Small sample size. Participants all were involved in various therapeutic programs in addition to the CE program or PT.
Reddihough et al. (1998)	To compare the effectiveness of a CE program compared with an NDT program for children with CP	Level I—Randomized control trial. *N* = 66 children with a definitive diagnosis of CP and varying cognitive ability, ages 12–36 mo Treatment CE program, *n* = 34 Control NDT program, *n* = 32	*Intervention* Participants attended individual therapy and a CE-based group. All participants received therapy in a clinic setting. Control: The participants in the NDT group had individual therapy and attended a play group with their caregiver. The CE participants averaged 2 hr, 48 min, of therapy per wk, and the NDT participants averaged 2 hr, 54 min, of therapy per wk. Duration was 6 mo. *Outcome Measures* • VAB • GMFM • Reynell Developmental Language Scale.	In relation to cognition, the control group (NDT) scored lower overall than the treatment group (CE). For language, organizational behaviors, and ADL function, the treatment group had significantly higher scores than the control group on the basis of caregiver ratings. Gross motor behaviors were also significantly higher for the treatment group.	The sample size of 66 was small, and the length of the intervention was relatively short (6 months). The study did not include a nontreatment group, and the control group received more hours of therapy on average than the treatment group.

http://dx.doi.org/10.1111/j.1469-8749.1998.tb12345.x

Context-Focused Intervention

Law et al. (2011)	To evaluate the efficacy of a child-focused vs. context-focused intervention in improving performance of functional tasks and mobility in young children with CP	Level 1—Randomized control trial. $N = 128$ children with Level I–V GMFCS level CP Child-focused group, $n = 71$, Mean age = 3.5 yr ($SD = 1.4$) Context-focused group, $n = 57$, Mean age = 3.9 yr ($SD = 1.4$)	*Intervention* Children received either a child-focused or a context-focused approach for 6 mo (18–24 sessions). In the child-focused group, occupational or physical therapists provided therapy to remediate the sensory or motor impairments and practice-specific movements and tasks. In the context-focused group, therapists focused on changing the constraints within the task, the environments that were constraining performance, or both. *Outcome Measures* • PEDI • Range of motion • GMFM • Preschool Children's Participation Scale.	The groups were similar at baseline. Both received equivalent amounts of therapy (18.7 child-focused and 17.7 context-focused therapy sessions). PEDI scores improved significantly, but the groups did not differ except for a small effect on the Caregiver Assistance Scales mobility subscale (child-focused group improved more). Change scores did not differ for GMFCS levels. GMFM scores improved for both groups. Participation improved in play intensity, physical activity intensity and diversity, and total score intensity (only). Children who received context-focused therapy made similar improvements to those who received child-focused therapy.	This study compared 2 interventions and lacked a control group. Neither therapy reflects typical intervention for children with CP.

http://dx.doi.org/10.1111/j.1469-8749.2011.03962.x

(Continued)

Table D.3. Evidence for Interventions Used in Occupational Therapy to Promote Motor Performance *(Cont.)*

Author/Year	Study Objectives	Level/Design/Participants	Intervention and Outcome Measures	Results	Study Limitations
Interventions to Promote Prewriting in Preschool Children With Visual–Motor Delays					
Case-Smith (2000a)	To examine how performance components and variables in intervention influenced fine motor and functional outcomes in preschool children	Level III—Pretest–posttest. $N = 44$ children ages 4–6 yr with fine motor delays	*Intervention* 22 collaborating OT practitioners provided direct intervention to the participants. Therapists weekly recorded their service delivery model, goals, and activities (e.g., sensory integration, motor–manipulation, self-care, play–peer interaction). *Outcome Measures* • 9-Hole Peg Test • Motor Accuracy test of the Sensory Integration and Praxis Test • Developmental Test of Visual Perception • PDMS Fine Motor Scale • Draw-a-Person • PEDI (Self-Care Function and Social Function).	The participants made statistically significant gains in all eight measures over the course of the academic year.	Explanations, rationale, and time were not given for activities and goals. Precise measurements of the OT sessions were not documented.
Dankert et al. (2003)	To examine the effectiveness of OT on enhancing visual–motor skills in preschool children	Level II—Quasi-experimental, two-factor mixed design. Preschool children with developmental delays, $n = 12$ Children without disabilities receiving OT and students without disability not receiving OT, $n = 15$ Age range = 3–6 yr	*Intervention* Individual and group OT intervention addressing visual–motor skills. *Outcome Measures* Visual–Motor Integration (Beery).	Results showed that students with developmental delays demonstrated statistically significant improvement in visual–motor skills and developed skills at a rate faster than expected compared with typically developing peers on the Visual Motor Integration.	The administrator of the assessments provided therapy and was not blinded to the study. Additional therapy was administered to children with developmental disabilities.

http://dx.doi.org/10.5014/ajot.57.5.542

Author/Year	Study Objectives	Level/Design/Participants	Intervention and Outcome Measures	Results	Study Limitations
Davies & Gavin (1994)	To compare the effectiveness of a group–consultative model of therapy with that of a direct model on preschool-age children with developmental delays	Level II—Nonrandomized controlled study. N = 18 children ages 3–5 yr. Intervention group, n = 10. Control program for children with disabilities, n = 8	*Intervention* Participants received both occupational and PT twice weekly. *Control:* Classroom staff members met with the occupational and physical therapists weekly for 30 min each. *Outcome Measures* • PDMS • Vineland Adaptive Behavior Scale • Central Institute for Deaf Preschool Performance Scales: nonverbal intelligence quotient.	Participants in both groups increased in fine and gross motor skills. The development rate of motor skills for all of the participants paralleled that of typically developing children. The scores on the VABS (except for daily living scales) were significantly increased for all participants.	Small sample size. Participants were from a specific geographical area, no nontreatment group, and no randomization.

http://dx.doi.org/10.5014/ajot.48.2.155

Author/Year	Study Objectives	Level/Design/Participants	Intervention and Outcome Measures	Results	Study Limitations
DeGangi et al. (1993)	To compare the benefits of a child-centered therapy approach emphasizing child-initiated play interactions within a structured therapy environment with those of therapist-directed, structured sensorimotor therapy approach	Level II—Repeated measures interventions (AB cross-over design) with randomization of the treatment interventions. N = 12 preschool children with sensory–motor dysfunction. Intervention A first, n = 6. Intervention B first, n = 6. Mean age = 53 mo	*Intervention* *Intervention A:* Child-centered sensorimotor therapy. *Intervention B:* Structured sensoryimotor therapy. *Outcome Measures* • PDMS • DeGangi–Berk Test of Sensory Integration • Touch Inventory for Preschoolers • Vineland Adaptive Behavior Scales • Child Behavior Checklist • McCarthy Scales of Children's Abilities.	Structured sensorimotor therapy was more useful than child-centered therapy in promoting gross motor skills, functional skills, and sensory integrative functions. Child-centered therapy appeared to promote fine motor skills better, but the difference was not statistically significant.	There was no control group. The sample size was small and similar in socioeconomic status. Different therapists were used to treat the children. Early intervention services continued throughout the study.

http://dx.doi.org/10.5014/ajot.47.9.777

Note. ADLs = activities of daily living; AROM = active range of motion; BiT = bimanual training; CE = conductive education; CI = constraint induced; CIMT = constraint-induced movement therapy; COPM = Canadian Occupational Performance Measure; CP = cerebral palsy; EBS = Emerging Behaviors Scale; GMFCS = Gross Motor Function Classification System; GMFM = Gross Motor Function Measure; MACS = Manual Ability Classification System; mCIMT = modified constraint-induced movement therapy; NDT = neurodevelopmental treatment; NICU = neonatal intensive care unit; NIDCAP = Newborn Individualized Developmental Care and Assessment Program; OT = occupational therapy; PDMS = Peabody Developmental Motor Scale; PEDI = Pediatric Evaluation of Disabilities Inventory; PFMS = Peabody Fine Motor Scales; PMAL = Pediatric Motor Activity Log; PROM = passive range of motion; PT = physical therapy; QUEST = Quality of Upper Extremity Skills Test; SD = standard deviation; TAUT = Toddler Arm Use Test; VAB = Vulpe Assessment Battery.

Suggested citation: Case-Smith, J., Frolek Clark, G. J., & Schlabach, T. L. (2013). Systematic review of interventions to promote motor performance for children ages 0–5 years. (Suppl. Table 1). *American Journal of Occupational Therapy, 67.*

Table D.4. Evidence for Occupational Therapy Interventions to Improve Cognitive Development

Author	Study Objectives	Level/Design/ Participants	Intervention and Outcome Measures	Results	Study Limitations
Barrera et al. (1991)	To determine the long-term effectiveness of an early intervention program with participants with high- and low-birth-weight preterm infants	Level I—Randomized control trial. $N = 67$ preterm and full-term children (follow-up at age 5 yr)	*Intervention* The initial study included 3 in-home groups: developmental programming intervention, parent–child intervention, and control group. *Outcome Measures* Various, including Minnesota Child Developmental Inventory.	Some significant differences were noted, but not in the cognitive area. Children with very low birth weight scored lower in the cognitive area as compared with other groups.	McCarthy Scale may underestimate developmental functioning. Study had small sample size.
http://dx.doi.org/10.1177/027112149101000403					
Brooks-Gunn et al. (1992)	To implement the Infant Health and Development Program in a low-birth-weight population through a center-based program focusing on cognitive functioning	Level I—Randomized control trial. $N = 985$ low-birth-weight preterm infants Intervention group $n = 377$ Control group $n = 608$	*Intervention* Intervention included home visits (weekly during Year 1 and biweekly during Years 2 and 3), child care at a child developmental center, and parent group meetings. *Outcome Measures* • BSID • Stanford-Binet Intelligence Scale • Peabody Picture Vocabulary Test–Revised • Visual Motor Integration Test.	Significant effects seen at 24 and 36 mo in cognitive domains. No significant differences were found for the BSID Motor Scale.	Patterns in ethnicity and level of education may skew results. Results cannot be generalized.
http://dx.doi.org/10.1016/S0022-3476(05)80896-0					
Gulsrud et al. (2007)	To examine the effect of intervention on affect, gaze, joint attention, behaviors, and verbalizations in children diagnosed with ASD	Level I—Randomized control trial. $N = 35$ children (ages 33–54 mo) diagnosed with autism Joint attention, $n = 17$ Symbolic play, $n = 18$	*Intervention* Joint attention and symbolic play interventions. *Outcome Measures* Eye gaze, affect, nonverbal gestures, and verbalization were coded.	Children in joint attention intervention improved in acknowledgment of novel objects.	Study had small sample size with few diverse participants.
http://dx.doi.org/10.1177/1362361307083255					

Study	Design	Intervention	Results	Limitations
Kleberg et al. (2002) To examine the effect of NIDCAP on the 1-yr development of infants born with a gestational age of < 32 wk	Level I—Randomized control trial. N = 20 premature infants NIDCAP group n = 11 Control group n = 9	*Intervention* Intervention group received care in the NICU according to the NIDCAP. Follow-up at 12 mo of adjusted age. *Outcome Measure* BSID	Cognitive development was significantly higher for experimental group; no significant difference on the Psychomotor Developmental Index.	Study had small sample size. NIDCAP program is a multidisciplinary dependent program with complex interventions (e.g., education, physical modifications). Higher proportion of girls in control group.
http://dx.doi.org/10.1016/S0378.3782(02)00014-2				
Maguire et al. (2009) To investigate the effect of NIDCAP on growth and cognitive, psychomotor, and neurodevelopment at ages 1 and 2 yr in infants born at < 32 wk gestational age	Level I—Randomized control trial. N = 168 premature infants recruited; 148 children assessed at age 1 yr (70 intervention, 78 control) and 146 children assessed at age 2 yr (68 intervention, 78 control)	*Intervention* Intervention group received care in the NICU according to the NIDCAP. Follow-up at 1 and 2 yr of corrected age. *Outcome Measures* Neurological outcome, Dutch BSID.	No statistically significant differences found between groups at 1- or 2-yr follow-up.	The intervention and control group infants were both cared for in the same unit so there may have been contamination in care. The intervention period was shorter than most NIDCAP programs.
http://dx.doi.org/10.1542/peds.2008-1950				
McCormick et al. (2006) To determine whether differences such as IQ and achievement would be observed in the Infant Health and Development Program, especially in the heavier low-birth-weight group at 18-yr follow-up	Level I—Randomized control trial. N = 638 individuals now age 18 who participated in a study for low-birth-weight preterm infants n = 382 children in the intervention program n = 226 in follow-up program	*Intervention* Educational program delivered through home visits, center-based program, and parent support groups. *Outcome Measures* • Woodcock–Johnson Tests of Achievement–Revised • Weschler Abbreviated Scale of Intelligence • Peabody Picture Vocabulary Test (PPVT)–Version III.	Experimental group had higher scores on the PPVT and math achievement. Scores on the cognitive testing approached significance.	Sample was too small to achieve statistical significance in adverse outcomes. There was a low response rate at this follow-up. Sample was not disadvantaged, so it was more difficult to detect differences in some areas.
http://dx.doi.org/10.1542/peds.2005-1316				

(*Continued*)

Table D.4. Evidence for Occupational Therapy Interventions to Improve Cognitive Development (*Cont.*)

Author	Study Objectives	Level/Design/ Participants	Intervention and Outcome Measures	Results	Study Limitations
Melnyk et al. (2001)	To evaluate the effectiveness of a parent-focused intervention program Creating Opportunities for Parent Empowerment (COPE) on infant cognitive development and maternal coping	Level I—Randomized control trial. *N* = 42 mothers (ages 18–38) of low-birth-weight premature infants hospitalized in a NICU Experimental group *n* = 20 Control group *n* = 22	*Intervention* COPE is an educational–behavioral program (educates mothers about physical characteristics and behaviors of low-birth-weight infant, interaction with infant, and activities to enhance development) in the NICU through 1 wk after discharge. *Outcome Measures* • BSID (Mental Development Index) • Assessment Feeding Scale • Home Observation for Measurement of the Environment.	Experimental group had significantly higher cognitive scores at 3 and 6 mo corrected age.	Limitations included small sample size; BSID–II being used for purposes other than its accurate prediction of normal IQs; and use of the Parental Beliefs Scale (baby subscale), which has low internal consistency reliability.
http://dx.doi.org/10.1002/nur.1038					
Nelson et al. (2001)	To evaluate the effects of CNS injury by comparing infants who had experienced either intraventricular hemorrhage or periventricular leukomalacia with extremely premature infants who did not experience CNS injury. The researchers also compared infants who received auditory–tactile–visual–vestibular intervention with those who did not.	Level I—Randomized control trial. *N* = 37 preterm infants with severe central nervous system injury or extreme prematurity	*Intervention* Multisensory (auditory–tactile–visual–vestibular) intervention in hospital until 2 mo corrected age. *Outcome Measures* • Dyadic Mutuality Code • Nursing Child Assessment Feeding Scale • Revised BSID.	No statistically significant difference between groups; however, experimental group had better motor and mental performance and had fewer cerebral palsy diagnoses at 1 yr. Infants with periventricular leukomalacia had significantly poorer mental development despite the group assignment.	Study had small sample size and lack of randomization associated with post hoc reconfiguration of groups based on type of brain injury. Length of intervention may have been too short to overcome serious neurodevelopmental disorders.

Author/Year	Study Objectives	Level/Design/Participants	Intervention and Outcome Measures	Results	Study Limitations
Olafsen et al. (2006)	To evaluate the effects of optimized neonatal mother–infant transactions on joint attention at 12 mo and to analyze whether an early intervention program to increase parents' sensitivity to infants' behaviors enhanced joint attention at 12 mo	Level I—Randomized control trial. $N = 140$ preterm infants, 75 term infants Intervention group, $n = 71$ (36 boys, 35 girls); Mean gestational age = 30 wk Control group $n = 69$ (37 boys, 32 girls); Mean gestational age = 30 wk Term infants, $n = 75$ (40 boys, 35 girls); Mean gestational age = 39 wk	*Intervention* The Vermont Intervention Program for Low Birth Weight Infants (Rauh, Achenbach, Nurcombe, Howell, & Teti, 1988), which emphasizes transition: parents appreciating their baby's specific behaviors and being sensitive to the infant's cues and teaching parents to respond to cues. Neonatal nurses met with the parents every day for 7 days before discharge. They made 4 home visits after discharge. *Outcome Measures* • The Early Social Communication Scales • Joint attention behaviors, behavioral requests, and social interaction behaviors were measured through behavioral counts from videotaped sessions.	Preterm intervention group was significantly higher in initiating joint attention and responding to social interaction. Term group scored moderately higher than the preterm control group. Infants did not show differences in responding to joint attention or responding to requests. Children's ability to integrate complex information may not be affected by this intervention.	Limited applicability to occupational therapists. Limited description of the intervention in the report.
http://dx.doi.org/10.1016/j.infbeh.2006.07.004					
Orton et al. (2009)	To examine the effects of early developmental intervention after discharge from the hospital on motor and cognitive development in preterm infants	Level I—Systematic review. Participants of each included study were infants born at < 37 wk gestational age with no major congenital abnormalities. 17 studies examined outcomes in infancy and school-age; 11 included in the meta-analysis.	*Intervention* Infant interventions to improve cognitive or motor outcomes, performed in the hospital, home, or community center. Goals included parent–infant relationships and infant development. *Outcome Measures* Outcomes assessed using motor or cognitive measures.	Early developmental interventions improved cognitive outcomes at infants' age and at preschool age. The results were not sustained at school age. Early intervention had little effect on motor outcomes. Benefits of developmental intervention may be restricted to short-term gains in cognitive outcomes.	Outcomes compiled were diverse; of 17 studies, only 9 had data analysis sufficient to include in the meta-analysis.
http://dx.doi.org/10.1111/j.1469-8749.2009.03414.x					

(Continued)

Table D.4. Evidence for Occupational Therapy Interventions to Improve Cognitive Development *(Cont.)*

Author	Study Objectives	Level/Design/ Participants	Intervention and Outcome Measures	Results	Study Limitations
Resnick et al. (1988)	To develop a preventative model of care for premature infants (under 1,800 g) and compare it with a traditional remedial method	Level I—Randomized control trial. *N* = 41 premature infants Experimental group *n* = 21 Control group *n* = 20	*Intervention* Preventative model vs. traditional remedial model. Preventative model included daily intervention in the NICU and twice monthly intervention in a home developmental program. Traditional remedial model included referral to intervention agencies, if needed, at 6-mo follow-up. *Outcome Measures* • BSID • Greenspan–Lieberman Observation Scale.	Statistically significant differences between groups on the BSID (Mental Development Index) found at 12 mo but not at 6 mo. No significant difference between groups on the Psychomotor Developmental index at 6- or 12-mo assessment.	Study had a small sample size of 41. Control for various interventions was not established, so it was difficult to identify specific interventions that were most effective.

http://dx.doi.org/10.1097/00004703-198804000-00004

Author	Study Objectives	Level/Design/ Participants	Intervention and Outcome Measures	Results	Study Limitations
Whalen et al. (2006)	To examine collateral changes in social initiations, positive affect, play, imitation, and language after participation of children with ASD in a joint attention training program	Level IV—Multiple baseline, single subject *N* = 4 children with ASD and 6 peer models Mean age = 4 yr, 2 mo	*Intervention* The joint attention treatment used naturalistic behavior modification techniques that included discrete trial training and pivotal response training. The child was taught to respond to joint attention bids, then was taught to initiate joint attention bids. *Outcome Measures* • Unstructured Joint Attention Assessment, rated in 30 min of play • Structured Joint Attention Assessment, rated in Structured Play, Empathic Response, and Structured Play Assessment • Play and language were measured in 10-min probes.	The 4 participants showed increases in social initiations and positive affect at posttreatment; 3 improved in empathic response. All improved on the Structured Play Assessment. Imitation increased an average of 20%. No changes in the rate of functional or symbolic play were found. Improved joint attention may lead to increased attention to social stimuli.	Study had small sample size. No standardized assessments were used.

http://dx.doi.org/10.1007/s10803-006-0108z

Author/Year	Study Objectives	Level/Design/Participants	Intervention and Outcome Measures	Results	Study Limitations
Wong et al. (2007)	To determine the effectiveness of symbolic play skills vs. joint attention skills with children diagnosed with autism	Level I—Randomized control trial. $N = 41$ children (ages 31–55 mo) diagnosed with autism Symbolic play, $n = 21$ Joint attention, $n = 20$	*Intervention* Joint attention and symbolic play interventions with applied behavior analysis were first taught at a table, then generalization was attempted during floor setting. *Outcome Measures* • Mullen Scales of Early Learning • Structured Play Assessment • Early Social Communication Skills Assessment.	Results were inconclusive and dependent on many factors. In general, children with autism mastered criteria at table setting before generalizing skills in floor play.	Study had small sample size with few diverse participants. Significant language differences existed between groups.

Note. ASD = autism spectrum disorder; BSID = Bayley Scales of Infant and Toddler Development; CNS = central nervous system; NICU = neonatal intensive care unit; NIDCAP = Newborn Individualized Developmental Care and Assessment Program.

This table is a product of AOTA's Evidence-Based Practice Project and the *American Journal of Occupational Therapy*. Copyright © 2013 by the American Occupational Therapy Association. It may be freely reproduced for personal use in clinical or educational settings as long as the source is cited. All other uses require written permission from the American Occupational Therapy Association. To apply, visit www.copyright.com.

Suggested citation: Frolek Clark, G. J., & Schlabach, T. L. (2013). Systematic review of occupational therapy interventions to improve cognitive development in children ages birth–5 years (Suppl. Table 1). *American Journal of Occupational Therapy, 67.*

Table D.5. Evidence for the Effectiveness of Different Service Delivery Models and Methods in Occupational Therapy Services for Young Children and Their Families

Author/Year	Study Objectives	Level/Design/ Participants	Intervention and Outcome Measures	Results	Study Limitations
Barlow et al. (2009)	To address whether group-based parenting programs are effective in improving maternal psychosocial health, including anxiety, depression, and self-esteem	Level I—Systematic review (Cochrane) 26 randomized control trials. Control as waiting-list, no-treatment, or placebo control group. *Criteria for programs:* Group-based format, structured program, variety of theoretical frameworks developed largely with the intention of helping parents to manage children's behavior and improve family functioning and relationships.	*Intervention* Group-based parenting programs: Behavioral, multimodal, humanistic, cognitive–behavioral, and rational–emotive therapy programs; maternal anxiety, depression, self-esteem. *Outcome Measures* Meta-analysis for 5 outcomes (depression, anxiety or stress, self-esteem, social support, relationship with spouse and marital adjustment).	All programs reviewed were successful in producing positive change in maternal psychosocial health. Meta-analyses showed statistically significant results favoring intervention groups for depression, anxiety or stress, self-esteem, and relationship with spouse and marital adjustment (not social support). Meta-analysis of follow-up data suggested continued improvement in self-esteem (significant), depression, and marital adjustment (not significant).	Some limitations regarding responses (e.g., 8 studies did not account for the number of parents who dropped out of the evaluation or were lost to follow-up).

					No reliability and validity reported for outcome measures.
Bierman et al. (2008)	To determine whether an intervention that focused on self-regulation (teaching children ways to calm down), emotional awareness, and social problem solving would lead to changes in executive function (EF) skills and school readiness	Level I—Randomized control trial. $N = 356$ children in 44 Head Start classrooms randomly assigned to an enriched intervention Head Start Research Based, Developmentally Informed (REDI) or to usual-practice classrooms. Assessments tracked the progress of 356 4-year-old children over the course of the prekindergarten year.	*Intervention* Included the Preschool PATHS Curriculum and components targeting language and emergent literacy skills. The intervention was delivered by classroom teachers, integrated into their ongoing classroom programs, including curriculum-based lessons, center-based extension activities, and training in coaching strategies to support generalized skill development. Extensive monitoring of program implementation indicated that teachers delivered the intervention with fidelity. *Outcome Measures* Cognitive and behavioral performance tasks, measures of school readiness, language and emergent literacy, and social–emotional regulation.	Preventive intervention fostered the development of executive regulatory systems; executive regulatory skills were promoted with strategic, classroom-level preventive intervention; the provision of intervention appeared particularly beneficial to children who started the year with low levels of behavioral inhibitory control. The support provided by REDI compensated for these EF deficits, promoting social–emotional competence and aggression control of less skillful children who struggled in usual-practice classrooms. The intervention effects on emergent literacy and social–emotional competencies noted highlight the potential of compensating for delays in EF skills associated with socioeconomic disadvantage, promoting EF skill development during the prekindergarten years to foster school readiness.	

http://dx.doi.org/10.1017/S0954579408000394

| Bruder (1997) | To examine the effects of different service delivery models on the development of toddlers with disabilities receiving EI within natural group environments | Level II—Two groups non-randomized cohort.

$N = 70$ toddlers with disabilities receiving EI services. | *Intervention*
Full- or part-time specialized instruction and therapy within or outside of the natural group setting.

Outcome Measures
Indices of child development and social competence; family background, needs, use of community resources, and social support; and the family's evaluation of their child's intervention program. Evaluations conducted every 3 mo, ages 24–36 mo. | Few strong relationships were found between service characteristics; no clear models of service delivery were identified. Service location and modality were most consistently related to child development. Services provided at the EI center, in a group environment, and using a consulting model correlated with greater motor and social–developmental change than the alternatives. | Nonrandomized with many potential service characteristic variables explored.

No control group. |

(Continued)

Table D.5. Evidence for the Effectiveness of Different Service Delivery Models and Methods in Occupational Therapy Services for Young Children and Their Families (Cont.)

Author/Year	Study Objectives	Level/Design/Participants	Intervention and Outcome Measures	Results	Study Limitations
Bruder (2003)	To investigate an alternative service delivery model for infants and toddlers eligible under Part C who are identified as English-language learners	Level II—Nonrandomized controlled intervention. $N = 19$ children, 9 boys, 10 girls; 11 households reported English spoken in the household, 8 households reported no English spoken in home; 8 families completed the data collection process in the intervention group. Intervention group $n = 10$ Control group $n = 9$	*Intervention:* Weekly child-based EI that focused on activities that occurred in the home or community likely to be interesting to the child. 24 wk long. *Outcome Measures* 30 outcome measures, including • Diagnostic reports • Family evaluation of intervention practices • Family Activity Setting Log • Activity Setting Observation Scale • Developmental Observation Checklist • Audiorecorded language samples.	90% of families reported that the Responsive Teaching Method was useful, effective, and did not disrupt their daily activities. Children in the control group had significantly higher levels of negative affect and significantly lower levels of child engagement. Control group parents showed significantly lower levels of parent effectiveness. The intervention group showed significantly higher levels of parent elaboration. The higher the child's interest in an activity, the greater the learning opportunities, child's engagement, child's competence, parent confidence, and parent competence. No significant differences were found between the intervention and control group in the child's overall development.	Small sample size. Questions regarding validity and reliability for outcome measures.
Chang et al. (2009)	To study the effects of parental involvement on parent and child outcomes	Level I—Randomized control trial. Longitudinal two-level hierarchical linear modeling. $N = 2,000$	*Intervention* 1,000 parents attending EHS and 1,000 parents not attending EHS parenting classes. *Outcome Measures* Parental cognitive stimulation and children's cognitive development measured on the Bayley II Mental Developmental Index.	Parents who attended parenting classes increased their children's cognitive and language stimulation over the years, engaged in more parent–child activities such as parent–child play and reading frequency, and had children with higher scores on the Bayley assessment.	Self-selected participants. Outcomes heavily reliant on self-reported data. Inconsistent randomization to groups. Problems with internal validity.

Citation	Purpose	Design/Level	Intervention & Outcome Measures	Results	Limitations
Chazan-Cohen et al. (2007)	To examine the impact of EHS on maternal depression, child cognition and language development, and child social–emotional development	Level I—Randomized controlled comparison. $N = 3{,}001$ families recruited from 17 federally funded EHS programs.	*Intervention* EHS program including home-based, center-based, and mixed programs. *Outcome Measures* • Maternal depression measured by the Center for Epidemiologic Studies Depression Scale • Children's cognitive and language development measured by the Bayley Scales of Infant Development, the MacArthur Communicative Development Inventories Short Form, and the Peabody Picture Vocabulary Test • Children's social–emotional development measured by the CBCL.	Two years after EHS, a statistically significant impact on maternal depression was found. Earlier initiation of EHS mediated the delayed impact on maternal depression.	Parent and therapist self-report measures for depressive symptoms may have influenced strength of some findings. Small sample size due to attrition and missing data.
Dunst et al. (2006)	To determine whether the different ways of conceptualizing natural learning environment EI practices had effects on parent and child functioning; in Study 1 (state study), to obtain a measure of the degree to which natural environments were used as contexts for practitioner-implemented interventions; in Study 2 (national study), to obtain a measure of degree to which everyday activities served as contexts for natural learning opportunities	Level II—Descriptive, survey-based comparisons of parents' responses and perceptions about two different service delivery methods.	*Intervention* Compared parent report on types of intervention: activity settings used as learning opportunities and EI implemented in activity settings. *Outcome Measures* • Perceived control appraisals • Perceived parenting competence • Perception of positive well-being • Perception of negative well-being • Perception of child progress.	*Study 1 (state study):* Everyday learning opportunities activities were associated with perceived control, parenting competence, positive parent well-being, and parents' judgment of child progress; the more EI was rated as implemented in everyday settings, the more attenuated positive well-being and the more heightened negative well-being. *Study 2 (national study):* In family activity settings, everyday learning opportunity activities were associated with positive consequences for perceived control, parenting competence, positive parent well-being, and parents' judgment of child progress.	Lack of clarity in defining intervention during Phase 1 Improvements may not have statistical significance.

http://dx.doi.org/10.1111/j1741-1130.2006.00047.x

(Continued)

Table D.5. Evidence for the Effectiveness of Different Service Delivery Models and Methods in Occupational Therapy Services for Young Children and Their Families *(Cont.)*

Author/Year	Study Objectives	Level/Design/Participants	Intervention and Outcome Measures	Results	Study Limitations
Dunst et al. (2007)	To examine relationship between the practice-based theory of family-centered help-giving and aspects of parent, family, and child behavior and functioning, considered relational help giving and participatory help giving	Level 1—Meta-analysis. *N* = 47 studies included if either or both relational or participatory dimensions of family-centered help-giving were assessed; one or more aspects of parent, family, or child behavior was measured; and the correlations between measures were reported or could be calculated from information in the research reports. Total number of study participants = 11,187; average sample size per study = 235; 89% of participants were mothers. Mean age across studies = 7–157 mo	*Intervention* The study participants were involved in or receiving services from EI programs, preschool special education programs, elementary schools, family support programs, mental health programs, neonatal intensive care units, specialty clinics, rehabilitation centers, or physician practices. *Outcome Measures* Self-efficacy beliefs, participant satisfaction, parenting behavior, personal and family well-being, social support, and child behavior.	The relationships between family-centered help-giving and outcomes were statistically significant in all six areas analyzed. Family-centered help-giving was hypothesized to be directly related to self-efficacy beliefs and parent, family, and child behavior and functioning and indirectly related to parent, family, and child behavior and functioning mediated by self-efficacy beliefs. Participatory help-giving (vs. relational help-giving) was strongly related to outcomes.	Relatively narrow participant background (mostly Caucasian mothers). Great range of emotional and other factors tied to various service settings (e.g., NICU vs. elementary school); findings could also indicate strength in the data. Majority of the studies included were correlational.

http://dx.doi.org/10.1002/mrdd.20176

Author/Year	Study Objectives	Level/Design/Participants	Intervention and Outcome Measures	Results	Study Limitations
Hume et al. (2005)	To examine the usage practices of EI and early childhood services and gauge the perceived outcomes and social validity of the specific interventions and methods of service delivery across the developmental domain	Level IV— Descriptive study that includes analysis of outcomes. $N = 195$ parents of 2- to 8-yr-old children with autism ($n = 141$), pervasive developmental disorder ($n = 32$), Asperger syndrome ($n = 17$), or other ($n = 6$) All participants were recruited through a database of a statewide resource center for autism; families originally volunteered to be in database; participants represented 50 of the 92 counties in the State of Indiana.	*Intervention* Questionnaire sent with specification to report only on services child received before kindergarten; parents given 4 wk to complete. *Outcome Measures* Types and amount of interventions used, strategies and curricular areas, settings, evaluation of service delivery, outcomes of interventions used.	Family members rated impact on developmental growth related to specific interventions. Parents strongly supported speech therapy, sensory integration, discrete trial training, and social supports. Parents rated their child's progress across 7 developmental areas and overall quality of life as a result of EI. Low positive correlations were found for consultative services and perceived cognitive outcomes; recreational therapy and perceived social outcomes; floor time and perceived social, speech, cognitive outcomes. Low negative correlations were found for behavior supports and perceived emotional outcomes; class aides and perceived adaptive skills. Highest correlation coefficient was between the use of regular progress reports and perceived quality of life outcomes; significant correlation coefficients were found between integration opportunities and the variables of perceived emotional, cognitive, speech, and quality-of-life outcomes.	Small and homogenous sample. Response bias. Statistical inconsistencies. Lack of reliability data for outcome measures.

http://dx.doi.org/10.1177/027112/14050250040101

(Continued)

Table D.5. Evidence for the Effectiveness of Different Service Delivery Models and Methods in Occupational Therapy Services for Young Children and Their Families (Cont.)

Author/Year	Study Objectives	Level/Design/Participants	Intervention and Outcome Measures	Results	Study Limitations
Lakes et al. (2009)	To examine the CUIDAR service delivery model in reducing disparities in access to and use of services and decreasing child behavior problems among low-income families	Level IV—Descriptive study with analysis; parent education course. *N* = 169 self-referred, low-income, predominantly minority families	*Intervention* Weekly sessions, community-based behaviorally oriented parent training curriculum with a child care component. Prevention and EI for children at risk for behavioral problems, via parent education. *Outcome Measures* • Demographics questionnaire • Pre- and posttreatment Strengths and Difficulties Questionnaire • Parent Satisfaction Questionnaire at the end of the program.	Potential barriers to service use: lack of insurance, limited knowledge about mental health services, administrative barriers, distrust of and unfamiliarity with service providers, and cultural-linguistic differences. Among Latinos, attendance rates are higher when services are provided in Spanish. Parents report improvements in overall child conduct problems, as well as high levels of satisfaction with the program.	Homogenous sample. Limited information on English proficiency and residency status of Latino families. Self-referred participants (may have missed extremely high-risk families). Did not directly measure parents' perceived barriers to participation in the CUIDAR model.
http://dx.doi.org/10.1177/1053815109331861					
Love et al. (2005)	To examine the impact of EHS programs on child and parenting outcomes	Level I—Randomized control trial. *N* = 3,001 families in EHS	*Intervention* Home- and center-based EHS curriculum. *Outcome Measures* • Cognition and language measured with the Bayley Scales of Infant Development and The Peabody Picture Vocabulary Test • Social–emotional development measured by the CBCL • Child health measured by survey • Parenting assessed with Home Observation for Measurement of the Environment.	Both home- and center-based approaches yielded greatest impact on child language development, child social–emotional development, and parenting behavior. No statistically significant impact for any outcomes with only center-based intervention. Children receiving only home-based approaches demonstrated higher levels of engagement during semistructured play; parents were rated as more supportive during semistructured play.	Small effect size. Small sample size for subgroups.
http://dx.doi.org/10.1037/0012-1649.41.6.885					

Study	Level/Design	Intervention / Outcome Measures	Results	Limitations
Luiselli et al. (2000) http://dx.doi.org/10.1177/136236130000400407	To determine whether intensity of service delivery, age at introduction of intervention, or both influenced developmental progress in 16 children with diagnoses of autism and pervasive developmental disorder who participated in home-based behavioral intervention	Level II—Retrospective analysis, two groups, non-randomized cohort study. Two age groups: < 3 yr old at start of intervention and > 3 yr old at start of intervention *Intervention* Home-based behavioral intervention. *Outcome Measures* Retrospective analysis of effects of home-based behavioral services by (Early) Learning Accomplishments Profile ([E]LAP).	Both groups demonstrated significant changes from pre- to posttreatment assessment for all 6 (E)LAP domains, but no significant difference in measures between the age groups for any of the domains. Duration of treatment was a predictor of change (significant for communication, cognition, and social–emotional domains).	Retrospective analysis with no control group and many external variables. Small sample size from a single therapy center.
McCart et al. (2009) http://dx.doi.org/10.1080/15240750902774692	To assess the feasibility and potential effectiveness of a family-based Multi-Tiered System of Support (MTSS) approach in an EHS setting Level III—Pilot study aimed at systematically studying the feasibility and effectiveness of an MTSS within a family support agency N = 30 families, with 13 completing a targeted intervention and 4 anticipated in the most intensive level	*Intervention* A universal intervention was implemented through a parenting program. *Outcome Measures* Included family stress.	Participants were satisfied with the service delivery and may have experienced reduced levels of stress as a result of their participation.	Small sample size. High attrition rate.
Moes & Frea (2002) http://dx.doi.org/10.1023/A:1021298729297	To determine how variables associated with the family context can be used to individualize Functional Communication Training (FCT) treatment packages and support family use of FCT in family routines Level IV—Multiple baseline. N = 3 families with children diagnosed with autism ages 3–5 yr	*Intervention* FCT in a home setting 2x/wk implemented by psychologist and behavior analysts. Contextual FCT (CFCT) followed traditional FCT. *Outcome Measures* Occurrence of problem behavior during observation sample; occurrence of functional communication during observation sample; parent report of sustainability of intervention packages; generalization outside of selected routines	*FCT:* Problem behavior decreased and functional communication increased when FCT was introduced into selected routines. No generalization outside of selected routines. *CFCT:* Problem behavior was extinguished or reduced to close to zero levels and functional communication increased during selected routines. Generalization occurred during nonroutine probes.	Small effect size. Reliance on self report. Attrition.

(Continued)

Table D.5. Evidence for the Effectiveness of Different Service Delivery Models and Methods in Occupational Therapy Services for Young Children and Their Families (Cont.)

Author/Year	Study Objectives	Level/Design/Participants	Intervention and Outcome Measures	Results	Study Limitations
Montgomery et al. (2009) http://dx.doi.org/10.1177/1053815198021020202	To review the effects of media-based cognitive–behavioral therapies for any young person with a behavioral disorder (diagnosed using a recognized instrument) compared with standard care and no-treatment controls	Level I—Systematic review (Cochrane). *N* = 11 studies including 943 parents of children with behavioral problems	*Intervention* Media-based treatment given to the parents of children with behavioral problems. *Outcome Measures* • Behavioral Assessment Scales • Composite Sleep Score • Child Behavior Checklist • Eyberg Child Behavior Inventory • Parent Daily Report • Preschool Behavior Questionnaire–Teacher Report.	Media-based interventions were found to have moderate, if variable, effect on child behavior problems (vs. no-treatment controls and as adjunct to medication). Significant improvements were made with the addition of up to 2 hr of therapist time. Most consistent effects were in mother's reports of child behavior.	No data collected in relation to type of media used for delivery. Limited participant data for socioeconomic status and culture.
Romer & Umbreit (1998)	To examine parent perceptions regarding family-centered service delivery (FCSD)	Level III—Nonrandomized, multiple baseline across participants. *N* = 9 families served by 3 service coordinators	*Intervention* FCSD *Outcome Measures* Family satisfaction survey.	High degree of satisfaction from parents when model was adequately implemented (85% or better); high degree of dissatisfaction when the model was not adequately implemented.	Small sample size. Low response rate.

VanLeit & Crowe (2002)	To determine the impact of an 8-wk occupational therapy intervention program for mothers of children with disabilities	Level I—Randomized control trial. $N = 38$ mothers of children with disabilities randomly assigned to a treatment or control group. No significant differences were found between the groups related to demographics. Employment ranged from 0–40 hr/wk, average level of education = 16 yr Mean age of mothers = 37	*Intervention* Individual and group sessions over 8-wk intervention period promoting increased satisfaction with time use and occupations. Occupational therapists led individual and group sessions in home and academic settings. *Outcome Measures* • COPM Satisfaction • COPM Performance • Time Perception Inventory • Time Use Analyzer.	Time Perception Inventory scores increased in both the treatment and the control groups. No significant change in Time Use Analyzer scores in either treatment or control group. Treatment group showed statistically significant increases in satisfaction scores on the COPM. No significant change occurred in performance scores on the COPM.	Design generally appropriate, but service delivery categories somewhat confusing. Difference between "early intervention implemented in activity settings (EI→AS)" vs. "activity settings used as sources of learning opportunities" (AS→EI)" difficult to ascertain; distinction dependent on parental reports of these characteristics. Percentage of returned surveys not provided, so representativeness of sample is unknown.

http://dx.doi.org/10.5014/ajot.56.4.402

(Continued)

Table D.5. Evidence for the Effectiveness of Different Service Delivery Models and Methods in Occupational Therapy Services for Young Children and Their Families (Cont.)

Author/Year	Study Objectives	Level/Design/Participants	Intervention and Outcome Measures	Results	Study Limitations
Whitaker (2002)	To determine parents' level of satisfaction with service provided and parental responses to different aspects of support offered as part of a local education authority (LEA) project in the United Kingdom, which provided support to the families of preschool children with autistic spectrum disorders and determine parents' experience of diagnosis and the families' needs in the immediate aftermath	Level III—Evaluation study with pre- and postprogram interviews. *N* = 18 families with preschool-age children who had received the diagnosis of autism spectrum disorder. A condition of the licensed use of the EarlyBird Program was the requirement to participate in this efficacy study by the National Autistic Society (NAS), including an evaluation interview; parental feedback on session-by-session basis.	*Intervention* In addition to enrollment in a LEA, families received a support worker who provided an ongoing home visiting service and delivered the NAS's EarlyBird package to help parents makes sense of their child and diagnosis; work with parents to develop skills to help their child's development; assist with management of challenging behavior; act as liaison and coordinate with other agencies and services; provide training and service development; 1x/wk (videotaped) in-home visits with 8 3-hr parent workshops interspersed with home visits. *Outcome Measures* On discharge from the program (around age 5), the mothers of all case-load children were interviewed with rating items and open-ended questions. Interviews were conducted by educational psychologists not involved in the service delivery.	Within 12 mo of finishing the program, all of the main components were rated *quite* or *very useful*; 3 parents rated the home visits *not very useful* and 1 parent found it somewhat invasive. All except 1 participant reported continuing to use the approaches learned in the program *quite often* or a *great deal*. Parents most frequently mentioned the information specific to autism and the practical intervention techniques as the most valuable part of the program. All parents rated the input of the support worker as *very useful* and with consistent themes emerging around making sense out of the child; theory in practice; and supporting care and education. Some parents expressed dissatisfaction with accessibility to information and resources after diagnosis.	No comparison group. Limited subgroup of participants with a very specific diagnosis.

http://dx.doi.org/10.1177/136236130200604007

Suggested citation: Kingsley, K., & Mailloux, Z. (2013). Evidence for the effectiveness of different service delivery models in early intervention services. (Suppl. Table 1). *American Journal of Occupational Therapy, 67.*

References

Aarts, P. B., Jongerius, P. H., Geerdink, Y. A., van Limbeek, J., & Geurts, A. C. (2010). Effectiveness of modified constraint-induced therapy in children with unilateral spastic cerebral palsy: A randomized controlled trial. *Neurorehabilitation and Neural Repair, 24,* 509–518. http://dx.doi.org/10.1177/1545968309359767

Aarts, P. B., Jongerius, P. H., Geerdink, Y. A., van Limbeek, J., & Geurts, A. C. (2011). Modified constraint-induced movement therapy combined with bimanual training (mCIMT–BiT) in children with unilateral spastic cerebral palsy: How are improvements in arm–hand use established? *Research in Developmental Disabilities, 32,* 271–279. http://dx.doi.org/10.1016/j.ridd.2010.10.008

Accreditation Council for Occupational Therapy Education. (2012). 2011 Accreditation Council for Occupational Therapy Education (ACOTE®) standards. *American Journal of Occupational Therapy, 66,* S6–S74. http://dx.doi.org/10.5014/ajot.2012.66S6

Achenbach, T. J. (2009). *The Achenbach System of Empirically Based Assessment (ASEDA): Development, findings, theory, and application.* Burlington: University of Vermont Research Center for Children, Youth, and Families.

Achenbach, T. M., McConaughy, S. H., & Howell, C. T. (1987). Child/adolescent behavioral and emotional problems: Implications of cross-informant correlations for situational specificity. *Psychological Bulletin, 101,* 213–232.

Agency for Healthcare Research and Quality, U.S. Preventive Services Task Force. (2009). *Standard recommendation language.* Retrieved February 14, 2009, from http://www.ahrq.gov/clinic/uspstf/standard.htm

Allik, H., Larsson, J. O., & Smedje, H. (2006). Sleep patterns of school-age children with Asperger syndrome or high-functioning autism. *Journal of Autism and Developmental Disorders, 36,* 585–595.

American Medical Association. (2012). *CPT 2013.* Chicago: Author.

American Occupational Therapy Association. (1979). Uniform terminology for occupational therapy. *Occupational Therapy News, 35,* 1–8.

American Occupational Therapy Association. (1989). Uniform terminology for occupational therapy (2nd ed.). *American Journal of Occupational Therapy, 43,* 808–815. http://dx.doi.org/10.5014/ajot.43.12.808

American Occupational Therapy Association. (1994). Uniform terminology for occupational therapy (3rd ed.). *American Journal of Occupational Therapy, 48,* 1047–1054. http://dx.doi.org/10.5014/ajot.48.11.1047

American Occupational Therapy Association. (1998). Standards of practice. *American Journal of Occupational Therapy, 52,* 866–869.

American Occupational Therapy Association. (2006). Policy 1.44: Categories of occupational therapy personnel. In *Policy manual* (2011 ed., pp. 33–34). Bethesda, MD: Author.

American Occupational Therapy Association. (2007). Specialized knowledge and skills in feeding, eating, and swallowing for occupational therapy practice. *American Journal of Occupational Therapy, 61,* 686–700. http://dx.doi.org/10.5014/ajot.61.6.686

American Occupational Therapy Association. (2008). Occupational therapy practice framework: Domain and process. *American Journal of Occupational Therapy, 56,* 609–639. http://dx.doi.org/10.5014/ajot.62.6.625

American Occupational Therapy Association. (2009). Guidelines for supervision, roles and responsibilities during the delivery of therapy services. *American Journal of Occupational Therapy, 63,* 779–803. http://dx.doi.org/10.5014/ajot.63.6.797

American Occupational Therapy Association. (2010). Standards of practice for occupational therapy. *American Journal of Occupational Therapy, 64,* S106–S111. http://dx.doi.org/10.5014/ajot.2010.64S106

American Occupational Therapy Association. (2011). Occupational therapy services in early childhood and school-based settings. *American Occupational Therapy Journal, 65*(Suppl.), S46–S54. http://dx/doi.org/10.5014/ajot.65S46

American Occupational Therapy Association. (2013). Guidelines for documentation of occupational therapy. *American Journal of Occupational Therapy, 67*(Suppl.).

Americans with Disabilities Act of 1990, Pub. L. 101–336, 42 U.S.C. § 12101.

Americans with Disabilities Act Amendments of 2008, Pub. L. 110-325, 122 Stat. 3553.

Anderson, S. E., & Whitaker, R. C. (2009). Prevalence of obesity among U.S. preschool children in different racial and ethnic groups. *Archives of Pediatrics and Adolescent Medicine, 163,* 344–348.

Arndt, S. W., Chandler, L. S., Sweeney, J. K., Sharkey, M. A., & McElroy, J. J. (2008). Effects of a neurodevelopmental treatment-based trunk protocol for infants with posture and movement dysfunction. *Pediatric Physical Therapy, 20,* 11–22. http://dx.doi.org/10.1097/PEP.0b013e31815e8595

Assistive Technology Act of 2004, Pub L. 108-364, 118 Stat. 1707–1737.

Ayres, A. J. (1989). *Sensory Integration and Praxis Tests.* Los Angeles: Western Psychological Services.

Barlow, J., Coren, E., & Stewart-Brown, S. (2009). Parent-training programmes for improving maternal psychosocial health. *Cochrane Database of Systematic Reviews, 2004,* CD002020.

Barlow, S. M., Finan, D. S., Lee, J., & Chu, S. (2008). Synthetic orocutaneous stimulation entrains preterm infants with feeding difficulties to suck. *Journal of Perinatology, 28,* 541–548. http://dx.doi.org/10.1038/jp200857

Barrera, M. E., Kitching, K. J., Cunningham, C. C., Doucet, D., & Rosenbaum, P. L. (1991). A 3-year early home intervention follow-up study with low birthweight infants and their parents. *Topics In Early Childhood Education, 10,* 14–28. http://dx.doi.org/10.1177/027112149101000403

Baum, C., & Christiansen, C. (2005). Outcomes: The results of intervenitons in occupational therapy practice. In C. H. Christianen & C. M. Baum (Eds.), *Occupational therapy performance, participation, and well-being* (pp. 523–534). Thorofare, NJ: Slack.

Bayley, N. (1993). *Bayley Scales of Infant Development Manual* (2nd ed.). San Antonio, TX: Psychological Corporation.

Bayley, N. (2005). *Bayley Scales of Infant and Toddler Development* (3rd ed.). San Antonio, TX: Psychological Corporation.

Beery, K., & Beery, N. (2010). *The Beery–Buktenica Developmental Test of Visual–Motor Integration* (6th ed.). San Antonio, TX: Pearson Assessments.

Benoit, D., Wang, E. E., & Zlotkin, S. H. (2000). Discontinuation of enterostomy tube feeding by behavioral treatment in early childhood: A randomized controlled trial. *Journal of Pediatrics, 137,* 498–503. http://dx.doi.org/10.1067/mpd.2000.108397

Berlin, K., Davies, H., Silverman, A., & Rudolph, C. (2009). Assessing family-based feeding strategies, strengths, and mealtime structure with the Feeding Strategies Questionnaire. *Journal of Pediatric Psychology, 34,* 1–10.

Berg, C., & LaVesser, P. (2006). The Preschool Activity Card Sort. *OTJR: Occupation, Participation and Health, 29,* 143–151.

Betz, A., Higbee, T. S., & Reagon, K. A. (2008). Using joint activity schedules to promote peer engagement in preschoolers with autism. *Journal of Applied Behavior Analysis, 41,* 237–241. http://dx.doi.org/10.1901/jaba.2008.41-237

Bier, J. A., Ferguson, A. E., Morales, Y., Liebling, J. A., Archer, D., Oh, W., & Vohr, B. R (1996). Comparison of skin-to-skin contact with standard contact in low-birth-weight infants who are breast-fed. *Archives of Pediatrics and Adolescent Medicine, 150,* 1265–1269. http://dx.doi.org/10.1001/archpedi.1996.02170370043006

Bierman, K. L., Nix, R. L., Greenberg, M. T., Blair, C., & Domitrovich, C. E. (2008). Executive functions and school readiness intervention: Impact, moderation, and mediation in the Head Start REDI program. *Development and Psychopathology, 20,* 821–843. http://dx.doi.org/10.1017/S0954579408000394

Black, M. M., Dubowitz, H., Hutcheson, J., Berenson-Howard, J., & Starr, R. H., Jr. (1995). A randomized clinical trial of home intervention for children with failure to thrive. *Pediatrics, 95,* 807–814.

Blanche, E. (2002). *Observations based on sensory integration theory.* Los Angeles: Western Psychological Corporation.

Blank, R., von Kries, R., Hesse, S., & von Voss, H. (2008). Conductive education for children with cerebral palsy: Effects on hand motor functions relevant to activities of daily living. *Archives of Physical Medicine and Rehabilitation, 89,* 251–259.

Blauw-Hospers, C. H., & Hadders-Algra, M. (2005). A systematic review of the effects of early intervention on motor development. *Developmental Medicine and Child Neurology, 47,* 421–432. http://dx.doi.org/10.1017/S0012162205000824

Boiron, M., Da Nobrega, L., Roux, S., Henrot, A., & Saliba, E. (2007). Effects of oral stimulation and oral support on non-nutritive sucking and feeding performance in preterm infants. *Developmental Medicine and Child Neurology, 49,* 439–444. http://dx.doi.org/10.1111/j.1469-8749.2007.00439.x

Bose, P., & Hinojosa, J. (2008). Reported experiences from occupational therapists interacting with teachers in inclusive early childhood classrooms. *American Journal of Occupational Therapy, 62,* 289–297. http://dx.doi.org/10.5014/ajot.62.3.289

Boyle, C. A., Boulet, S., Schieve, L. A., Cohen, R. A., Blumberg, S. J., Yeargin-Allsopp, M., . . . , Kogan, M. D. (2011). Trends in the prevalence of developmental disabilities in U.S. children, 1997–2008. *Pediatrics, 127,* 1034–1042.

Bragelien, R., Rokke, W., & Markestad, T. (2007). Stimulation of sucking and swallowing to promote oral feeding in premature infants. *Acta Paediatrica, 96,* 1430–1432. http://dx.doi.org/10.1111/j.1651-2227.2007.00448.x

Bricker, D., Pretti-Frontczak, K., & McComas, N. (1998). *An activity-based approach to early intervention.* Baltimore: Paul H. Brookes.

Bricker, D., & Waddell, M. (2002a). *Assessment, Evaluation and Programming System for Infants and Children* (2nd ed.). Baltimore: Paul H. Brookes.

Bricker, D., & Waddell, M. (2002b). *Assessment, Evaluation and Programming System for Three to Six Years* (2nd ed.). Baltimore: Paul H. Brookes.

Brooks-Gunn, J., Liaw, F. R., & Klebanov, P. K. (1992). Effects of early intervention on cognitive function of low birth weight preterm infants. *Journal of Pediatrics, 120,* 350–359. http://dx.doi.org/10.1016/S0022-3476(05)80896-0

Brown, T., & Burns, S. (2001). The efficacy of neurodevelopmental treatment in paediatrics: A systematic review. *British Journal of Occupational Therapy, 54,* 235–244.

Bruder, M. B. (1997). *An analysis of the effectiveness of staffing patterns for young children attending natural group environments for early intervention.* Washington, DC: U.S. Department of Education, Office of Educational Research and Improvement.

Bruder, M. B. (2003). *An examination of an alternative early intervention service delivery model for Latino families whose children are English language learners.* Washington, DC: U.S. Department of Education Office of Educational Research and Improvement.

Bruininks, R. H., & Bruininks, B. D. (2005). *Bruininks–Oseretsky Test of Motor Proficiency* (2nd ed.). Circle Pines, MN: American Guidance Service.

Bruininks, R. H., Woodcock, R. W., Weatherman, R. F., & Hill, B. K. (1996). *Scale of Independence Behavior–Revised.* Itasca, IL: Riverside.

Bundy, A. (1995). Assessment and intervention in school-based practice: Answering questions and minimizing discrepancies. In I. Ewen (Ed.), *Occupational and physical therapy in educational environments* (pp. 68–88). Binghamton, NY: Haworth Press.

Byars, K. C., Burklow, K. A., Ferguson, K., O'Flaherty, T., Santoro, K., & Kaul, A. (2003). A multicomponent behavioral program for oral aversion in children dependent on gastrostomy feedings. *Journal of Pediatric Gastroenterology and Nutrition, 37,* 473–480. http://dx.doi.org/10.1097/00005176-200310000-00014

Caldwell, B., & Bradley, R. (2001). *HOME Inventory administration manual.* Little Rock: University of Arkansas School of Medical Sciences.

Campbell, S. B. (1995). Behavior problems in preschool children: A review of recent research. *Journal of Child Psychology and Psychiatry and Allied Disciplines, 36,* 113–149.

Campbell, S. K. (1997). Therapy programs for children that last a lifetime. *Physical and Occupational Therapy in Pediatrics, 17,* 1–15.

Candler, C., Clark, G., & Swinth, Y. (2008). School-based services: What does OT bring to the IFSP and IEP table? *Journal of Occupational Therapy, Schools and Early Intervention, 1,* 17–24.

Carrasco, R., Skees-Hermes, S., Clark, G., Polichino, J., Ralabate, P., Thomas, L., . . . , Hughes, T. (2007). Occupational therapy service delivery to support child and family participation in context. In L. Jackson (Ed.), *Occupational therapy services for children and youth under IDEA* (3rd ed., pp. 89–128). Bethesda, MD: AOTA Press.

Case-Smith, J. (2000a). Effects of occupational therapy services on fine motor and functional performance in preschool children. *American Journal of Occupational Therapy, 54,* 372–380. http://dx.doi.org/10.5014/ajot.54.4.372

Case-Smith, J. (2000b). Self-care strategies for children with developmental disabilities. In C. Christiansen (Ed.), *Ways of living: Self-care strategies for special needs* (pp. 81–121). Bethesda, MD: AOTA Press.

Case-Smith, J. (2005). Development of childhood occupations. In J. Case-Smith (Ed.), *Pediatric occupational therapy and early intervention* (pp. 56–83). Woburn, MA: Butterworth-Heinemann.

Case-Smith, J. (2010). Development of childhood occupations. In J. Case-Smith (Ed.), *Occupational therapy for children* (6th ed., pp. 56–83). Maryland Heights, MO: Mosby.

Casto, G., & Mastropieri, M. A. (1986). The efficacy of early intervention programs: A meta-analysis. *Exceptional Children, 52,* 417–424.

Catanese, A., Coleman, G., King, J., & Reddihough, D. (1995). Evaluation of an early childhood programme based on principles of conductive education: The Yooralla project. *Child Health, 31,* 418–422.

Cauthen, N., & Fass, S. (2009). *Ten important questions about poverty and family economic hardship.* Retrieved April 13, 2012, from http://www.nccp.org/publications/pub_829.html

Centers for Disease Control and Prevention. (2012a). *Basic facts about childhood obesity.* Retrieved April 13, 2012, from http://www.cdc.gov/obesity/childhood/basics.html

Centers for Disease Control and Prevention. (2012b). *CDC growth charts.* Retrieved April 13, 2012, from http://www.cdc.gov/growthcharts/cdc_charts.htm/

Centers for Disease Control and Prevention. (n.d.). *A health care professional presentation: Learn the signs.* Retrieved April 13, 2012, from http://www.cdc.gov/ncbddd/actearly/hcp/index.html

Chandler, B. (2010). Introduction. In B. Chandler (Ed.), *Early childhood: Occupational therapy services for children birth to five* (p. 145). Bethesda, MD: AOTA Press.

Chang, M., Park, B., & Kim, S. (2009). Parenting classes, parenting behavior, and child cognitive development in Early Head Start: A longitudinal model. *School Community Journal, 19,* 155–174.

Chatoor, I., Hirsch, R., & Persinger, M. (1997). Facilitating internal regulation of eating: A treatment model for infantile anorexia. *Infants and Young Children, 9,* 12–22. http://dx.doi.org/10.1097/00001163-199704000-00004

Chazan-Cohen, R., Ayoub, C., Pan, B. A., Roggman, L., Raikes, H., & McKelvey, L., . . . Hart, A. (2007). *It takes time: Impacts of Early Head Start that lead to reductions in maternal depression two years later.* Lincoln: University of Nebraska, Department of Child, Youth, and Family Studies.

Chiarello, L. A., & Palisano, R. J. (1998). Investigation of the effects of a model of physical therapy on mother–child interactions and the motor behaviors of children with motor delay. *Physical Therapy, 78,* 180–194.

Child Abuse Prevention and Treatment Act (CAPTA), as amended by Pub. L. 111-320, the CAPTA Reauthorization Act of 2010.

Clark, G. F. (2010). Evaluation, assessment and outcomes in early childhood. In B. Chandler (Ed.), *Early childhood: Occupational therapy services for children birth to five* (pp. 131–178). Bethesda, MD: AOTA Press.

Clark, G. F., & Coster, W. (1998). Evaluation/problem solving and program evaluation. In J. Case-Smith (Ed.), *Occupational therapy: Making a difference in school system practice* (pp. 1–46). Bethesda, MD: AOTA Press.

Colarusso, R., & Hammill, D. (2003). *Motor-Free Visual Perception Test* (3rd ed.). Novato, CA: Academic Therapy Publications.

Coleman, G., King, J., & Reddihough, D. (1995). A pilot evaluation of conductive education-based intervention for children with cerebral palsy: The Tongala project. *Journal of Paediatrics and Child Health, 31,* 412–417.

Combating Autism Act of 2006, P. L. 109–416, 120 Stat. 2821.

Constantino, J., & Gruber, C. (2005). *The Social Responsiveness Scale*. Los Angeles: Psychological Corporation.

Crozier, S., & Tincani, M. (2007). Effects of social stories on prosocial behavior of preschool children with autism spectrum disorders. *Journal of Autism and Developmental Disorders, 37,* 1803–1814. http://dx.doi.org/10.1007/s10803-006-0315-7

Dankert, H. L., Davies, P. L., & Gavin, W. J. (2003). Occupational therapy effects on visual–motor skills in preschool children. *American Journal of Occupational Therapy, 57,* 542–549. http://dx.doi.org/10.5014/ajot.57.5.542

Daunhauer, L. A., Coster, W. J., Tickle-Degnen, L., & Cermak, S. A. (2007). Effects of caregiver-child interactions on play occupations among young children institutionalized in Eastern Europe. *American Journal of Occupational Therapy, 61,* 429–440. http://dx.doi.org/10.5014/ajot.61.4.429

Davies, P. L., & Gavin, W. J. (1994). Comparison of individual and group/consultation treatment methods for preschool children with developmental delays. *American Journal of Occupational Therapy, 48,* 155–161. http://dx.doi.org/10.5014/ajot.48.2.155

DeGangi, G. A., Wietlisbach, S., Goodin, M., & Scheiner, N. (1993). A comparison of structured sensorimotor therapy and child-centered activity in the treatment of preschool children with sensorimotor problems. *American Journal of Occupational Therapy, 47,* 777–786. http://dx.doi.org/10.5014/ajot.47.9.777

DeLuca, S. C., Echols, K., Law, C. R., & Ramey, S. L. (2006). Intensive pediatric constraint-induced therapy for children with cerebral palsy: Randomized, controlled, crossover trial. *Journal of Child Neurology, 21,* 931–938. http://dx.doi.org/10.1177/08830738060210110401

Dinnebeil, L., McInerney, W., Roth, J., & Ramasway, V. (2001). Itinerant early childhood special education services: Service delivery in one state. *Journal of Early Intervention, 24,* 35–44.

Dodge, D., Heroman, C., Colker, L., & Bickart, T. (2010). *Creative curriculum for preschoolers*. Washington, DC: Teaching Strategies.

Dodge, D., Rudick, S., & Berke, K. (2011). *Creative curriculum for infants, toddlers and twos*. Washington, DC: Teaching Strategies.

Dunlap, G., Lewis, T., & McCart, A. (2006). Program-wide positive behavior support for young children. *PSIB Newsletter, 3*(3). Retrieved April 13, 2012, from: http://www.pbis.org/pbis_newsletter/volume_3/issue3.aspx

Dunn, W. (1999). *The Sensory Profile: User's manual*. San Antonio, TX: Psychological Corporation.

Dunn, W. (2000). *Best practice in occupational therapy in community based services with children and families*. Thorofare, NJ: Slack.

Dunn, W. (2002). *Infant/Toddler Sensory Profile manual*. San Antonio, TX: Psychological Corporation.

Dunn, W. (2006). *Sensory Profile School Companion*. San Antonio, TX: Psychological Corporation.

Dunn, W., McClain, L., Brown, C., & Youngstrom, M. J. (1998). The ecology of human performance. In M. E. Neistadt & E. B. Creapeu (Eds.), *Willard and Spackman's occupational therapy* (9th ed., pp. 525–535). Philadelphia: Lippincott Williams & Wilkins.

Dunst, C. (2002). Family-centered practices: Birth through high school. *Journal of Special Education, 36,* 139–149.

Dunst, C. J., Bruder, M. B., Trivette, C. M., & Hamby, D. W. (2006). Everyday activity settings, natural learning environments, and early intervention practices. *Journal of Policy and Practice in Intellectual Disabilities, 3,* 3–10. http://dx.doi.org/10.1111/j.1741-1130.2006.00047.x

Dunst, C. J., Trivette, C. M., & Hamby, D. W. (2007). Meta-analysis of family-centered helpgiving practices research. *Mental Retardation and Developmental Disabilities Research Reviews, 13,* 370–378. http://dx.doi.org/10.1002/mrdd.20176

Durand, V. (1998). *Sleep better: A guide to improving sleep for children with special needs.* Baltimore: Paul H. Brookes.

Early Intervention Program for Infants and Toddlers with Disabilities, 76 Fed. Reg. 60, 140 (September 28, 2011), codified at 34 C.F.R. § 303.

Ecker, C., & Parham, L. D. (2010). *Sensory Processing Measure–Preschool Home Form.* Torrance, CA: West Psychological Services.

Education for All Handicapped Children Act of 1975, Pub. L. 94-142, 20 U.S.C. § 1400, *et seq.*

Einarsson-Backes, L. M., Deitz, J., Price, R., Glass, R., & Hays, R. (1994). The effect of oral support on sucking efficiency in preterm infants. *American Journal of Occupational Therapy, 48,* 490–498. http://dx.doi.org/10.5014/ajot.48.6.490

Epstein, A., & Hohmann, M. (2012). *The High-Scope Preschool Curriculum.* Ypsilanti, MI: High Scope Press.

Erhardt, R. (1990). *The Erhardt Developmental Vision Assessment* (2nd ed.). Maplewood, MN: Erhardt Developmental Products.

Erhardt, R. (1994). *Erhardt Developmental Prehension Assessment* (2nd ed.). Maplewood, MN: Erhardt Developmental Products.

Escalona, A., Field, T., Singer-Strunck, R., Cullen, C., & Hartshorn, K. (2001). Brief Report—Improvements in the behavior of children with autism following massage therapy. *Journal of Autism and Developmental Disorders, 31,* 513–516. http://dx.doi.org/10.1023/A:1012273110194

Farooqi, A., Hägglöf, B., Sedin, G., & Serenius, F. (2011). Impact at age 11 years of major neonatal morbidities in children born extremely preterm. *Pediatrics, 127,* e1247–e1257. http://dx.doi.org/10.1542/peds.2010-0806

Field, T., Field, T., Sanders, C., & Nadel, J. (2001). Children with autism display more social behaviors after repeated imitation sessions. *Autism, 5,* 317–323. http://dx.doi.org/10.1177/1362361301005003008

Fisher, A. (2006). Overview of performance skills and client factors. In H. Pendleton & W. Schultz-Krohn (Eds.), *Pedretti's occupational therapy: Practice skills for physical dysfunction* (pp. 372–402). St. Louis, MO: Mosby/Elsevier.

Fisher, A., Bryze, K., Hume, V., & Griswold, L. (2005). *School AMPS: School Version of the Assessment of Motor and Process Skills* (2nd ed.). Fort Collins, CO: Three Star Press.

Folio, R., & Fewell, R. (2000). *Peabody Developmental Motor Scales* (2nd ed.). Austin, TX: Pro-Ed.

Foss, J. (2010). Models and process of service provision in early childhood. In B. Chandler (Ed.), *Early childhood: Occupational therapy services for children birth to five* (pp. 109–129). Bethesda, MD: AOTA Press.

Fraser, K., Wallis, M., & St. John, W. (2004). Improving children's problem eating and mealtime behaviours: An evaluative study of a single session parent education. *Health Education Journal, 63,* 229–241. http://dx.doi.org/10.1177/001789690406300304

Fucile, S., Gisel, E., & Lau, C. (2002). Oral stimulation accelerates the transition from tube to oral feeding in preterm infants. *Journal of Pediatrics, 141,* 230–236. http://dx.doi.org/10.1067/mpd.2002.125731

Fucile, S., Gisel, E. G., & Lau, C. (2005). Effect of an oral stimulation program on sucking skill maturation of preterm infants. *Developmental Medicine and Child Neurology, 47,* 158–162. http://dx.doi.org/10.1017/S0012162205000290

Gaebler, C. P., & Hanzlik, J. R. (1996). The effects of a prefeeding stimulation program on preterm infants. *American Journal of Occupational Therapy, 50,* 184–192. http://dx.doi.org/10.5014/ajot.50.3.184

Garcia Coll, C. T., Halpern, L., Seifer, R., Meyer, E. C., Kilis, E., Lester, B. M., . . . Oh, W. (1996). Behavioral intervention and post-natal growth in full-term intrauterine growth retarded (IUGR) infants. *Early Human Development, 46,* 105–116. http://dx.doi.org/10.1016/0378-3782(96)01748-3

Giangreco, M., Cloninger, C., & Iverson, V. (2011). *Choosing Outcomes and Accommodations for Children (COACH): A guide to educational planning for students with disabilities* (3rd ed.). Baltimore: Paul H. Brookes.

Gioia, G., Espy, K., & Isquith, P. (2003). *Behavior Rating Inventory of Executive Function-Preschool Version.* Odessa, FL: Psychological Assessment Resources.

Girolami, G., & Campbell, S. (1994). Efficacy of a neurodevelopmental treatment program to improve motor control in infants born prematurely. *Pediatric Physical Therapy, 6,* 175–184.

Gisel, E. G., Tessier, M. J., Lapierre, G., Seidman, E., Drouin, E., & Filion, G. (2003). Feeding management of children with severe cerebral palsy and eating impairment: An exploratory study. *Physical and Occupational Therapy in Pediatrics, 23,* 19–44.

Glover, M. E., Preminger, J., & Sanford, A. (2002). *Early Learning Accomplishment Profile for Developmentally Young Children* (3rd ed.). Chapel Hill, NC: Chapel Hill Training-Outreach Project.

Gray, J. M. (1998). Putting occupation into practice: Occupation as ends, occupation as means. *American Journal of Occupational Therapy, 52,* 354–364.

Greer, A. J., Gulotta, C. S., Masler, E. A., & Laud, R. B. (2008). Caregiver stress and outcomes of children with pediatric feeding disorders treated in an intensive interdisciplinary program. *Journal of Pediatric Psychology, 33,* 612–620. http://dx.doi.org/10.1093/jpepsy/jsm116

Griffiths, R. (1996) *Griffiths Mental Development Scales–Revised: Birth to 2 years (GMDS 0–12).* Oxford, UK: Hogrefe.

Gulsrud, A. C., Kasari, C., Freeman, S., & Paparella, T. (2007). Children with autism's response to novel stimuli while participating in interventions targeting joint attention or symbolic play skills. *Autism, 11,* 535–546. http://dx.doi.org/10.1177/1362361307083255

Guralnick, M. J., Connor, R. T., Neville, B., & Hammond, M. A. (2006). Promoting the peer-related social development of young children with mild developmental delays: Effectiveness of a comprehensive intervention. *American Journal of Mental Retardation, 111,* 336–356. http://dx.doi.org/10.1352/0895-8017(2006)111[336:PTPSDO]2.0.CO;2

Gutstein, S. E., Burgess, A. F., & Montfort, K. (2007). Evaluation of the relationship development intervention program. *Autism, 11,* 397–411.

Hake-Brooks, S. J., & Anderson, G. C. (2008). Kangaroo care and breastfeeding of mother-preterm infant dyads 0–18 months: A randomized, controlled trial. *Neonatal Network, 27,* 151–159. http://dx.doi.org/10.1891/0730-0832.27.3.151

Haley, S., Coster, W., Ludlow, L., Haltiwanger, J., & Andrellos, P. (1992). *Pediatric Evaluation of Disability Inventory.* San Antonio, TX: Psychological Corporation.

Hamilton, B. E., Martin, J. A., & Ventura, S. J. (2011). Births: Preliminary data for 2010. *National Vital Statistics Reports, 60*(2). Hyattsville, MD: National Center for Health Statistics.

Hammill, D., Pearson, N., & Voress, J. (1993). *Developmental Test of Visual Perception* (3rd ed.). Austin, TX: Pro-Ed.

Handley-Moore, D., & Chandler, B. (2007). Occupational therapy decision-making process. In L. Jackson (Ed.), *Occupational therapy services for children and youth under IDEA* (3rd ed., pp. 59–87). Bethesda, MD: AOTA Press.

Hanft, B., & Pilkington, K. (2000). Therapy in natural environments: The means or end goal for early intervention. *Infants and Young Children, 12,* 1–13.

Hanft, B., Rush, D., & Shelden, M. (2004). *Coaching families and colleagues in early childhood.* Baltimore: Paul H. Brookes.

Hardin, B., & Peisner-Feinberg, E. (2004). *Learning Accomplishment Profile (3rd ed.; LAP–3) manual.* Chapel Hill, NC: Kaplan Early Learning Co.

Harms, T., Clifford, R., & Cryer, D. (2005). *The Early Childhood Environment Rating Scale–Revised.* New York: Teachers College Press.

Harrison, P., & Oakland, T. (2003). *Adaptive Behavior Assessment System, 2nd edition: Manual.* San Antonio: TX: Psychological Corporation.

Haywood, P. & McCann, J. (2009). A brief group intervention for young children with feeding problems. *Clinical Child Psychology and Psychiatry, 14,* 361–372. http://dx.doi.org/10.1177/1359104509104046

Henderson, A. (2006). Self-care and hand skills. In A. Henderson & C. Pehoski (Eds.), *Hand function in the child: Foundations for remediation* (pp. 193–216). St. Louis, MO: Mosby.

High Scope. (2002). *HighScope Child Observation Record (COR) for Infants and Toddlers.* Ypsilanti, MI: High Scope Press

Hinojosa, J., & Foto, M. (2004). Occupational therapy for documentation for reimbursement: Sensory integration. *Sensory Integration Special Interest Section Quarterly, 27,* 1–3.

Holloway, E. (1998). Early emotional development and sensory processing. In J. Case-Smith (Ed.), *Pediatric occupational therapy and early intervention* (pp. 163–197). Woburn, MA: Butterworth-Heinemann.

Holloway, E., & Chandler, B. (2010). Family-centered practice: It's all about relationships. In B. Chandler (Ed.), *Early childhood: Occupational therapy services for children birth to five* (pp. 77–107). Bethesda, MD: AOTA Press.

Honomichl, R. D., Goodlin-Jones, B. L., Burnham, M., Gaylor, E., & Anders, T. F. (2002). Sleep patterns of children with pervasive developmental disorders. *Journal of Autism and Developmental Disorders, 32,* 553–561.

Hovi, P., Andersson, S., Eriksson, J. G., Järvenpää, A. L., Strang-Karlsson, S., Mäkitie, O., & Kajantie, E. (2007). Glucose regulation in young adults with very low birth weight. *New England Journal of Medicine, 356,* 2053–2063.

Howard, J., Greyrose, E., Kehr, K., Espinosa, M., & Beckwith, L. (1996). Teacher-facilitated microcomputer activities: Enhancing social play and affect in young children with disabilities. *Journal of Special Education Technology, 13,* 36–47.

Hresko, W., Miguel, S., Sherbenou, R., & Burton, S. (1998). *Developmental Observation Checklist System (DOCS).* Austin, TX: Pro-Ed.

Hume, K., Bellini, S., & Pratt, C. (2005). The usage and perceived outcomes of early intervention and early childhood programs for young children with autism spectrum disorder. *Topics in Early Childhood Special Education, 25*, 195–207. http://dx.doi.org/10.1177/02711214050250040101

Humphry, R (1989). Early intervention and the influence of the occupational therapist on the parent-child relationship. *American Journal of Occupational Therapy, 43*, 738–742. http://dx.doi.org/10.5014.ajot/43.11.738

Hur, J., (1997). Skills for independence for children with cerebral palsy: A comparative longitudinal study. *International Journal of Disability, Development, and Education, 44*, 263–275.

Hwang, B., & Hughes, C. (2000). The effects of social interactive training on early social communicative skills of children with autism. *Journal of Autism and Developmental Disorders, 30*, 331–343. http://dx.doi.org/10.1023/A:1005579317085

Improving Head Start for School Readiness Act of 2007, Pub L. 110-134, 121 Stat. 1363, 42 U.S.C. 9801 *et seq.*

Individuals With Disabilities Education Act of 1997, Pub. L. 108–446, 20 U.S.C. § 1400 *et seq.*

Individuals with Disabilites Education Improvement Act of 2004, Part C regulations, 34 CFR Part 303 (2011).

Innocenti, M. S., & White, K. R., (1993). Are more intensive early intervention programs more effective? A literature review. *Exceptionality, 4*(1), 31–50.

Jackson, L. (Ed.). (2007). *Occupational therapy services for children and youth under IDEA* (3rd ed.). Bethesda, MD: AOTA Press.

Jadcherla, S. R., Stoner, E., Gupta, A., Bates, D. G., Fernandez, S., Di Lorenzo, C., & Linscheid, T. (2009). Evaluation and management of neonatal dysphagia: Impact of pharyngoesophageal motility studies and multidisciplinary feeding strategy. *Journal of Pediatric Gastroenterology and Nutrition, 48*, 186–192. http://dx.doi.org/10.1097/MPG.0b013e3181752ce7

Johnson-Martin, N., Attermeier, S., & Hacker, B. (2004a). *The Carolina Curriculum for Infants and Toddlers with Special Needs* (3rd ed.). Baltimore: Paul H. Brookes.

Johnson-Martin, N., Attermeier, S., & Hacker, B. (2004b). *The Carolina Curriculum for Preschoolers with Special Needs* (2nd ed.). Baltimore: Paul H. Brookes.

Karoly, L., Kilburn, R., & Cannon, J. (2005). *Children at risk: Consequences for school readiness and beyond.* Santa Monica, CA: RAND Corporation.

Kasari, C., Freeman, S., & Paparella, T. (2006). Joint attention and symbolic play in young children with autism: A randomized controlled intervention study. *Journal of Child Psychology and Psychiatry, and Allied Disciplines, 47*, 611–620. http://dx.doi.org/10.1111/j.1469-7610.2005.01567.x

Katz, L. (2010). STEM in the early years. *Early Childhood Research and Practice*, 1–7. Retrieved from http://ecrp.uiuc.edu/beyond/seed/katz.html

Kerwin, M. E. (1999). Empirically supported treatments in pediatric psychology: Severe feeding problems. *Journal of Pediatric Psychology, 24*, 193–214; discussion 215–196.

Kim, A., Vaughn, S., Elbaum, G., Hughes, M. T., Sloan, C. V., & Sridhar, D. (2003). Effects of toys or group composition for children with disabilities: A synthesis. *Journal of Early Intervention, 25*, 189–205. http://dx.doi.org/10.1177/105381510302500304

King, G., Law, M., King, S., Hurley, P., Rosenbaum, P., Janna, S., . . . Young, N. (2005). *Children's Assessment of Participation and Enjoyment (CAPE) and Preferences for Activities of Children (PAC)*. San Antonio, TX: Harcourt.

Kleberg, A., Westrup, B., Stjernqvist, K., & Lagercrantz, H. (2002). Indications of improved cognitive development at one year of age among infants born very prematurely who received care based on the Newborn Individualized Developmental Care and Assessment Program (NIDCAP). *Early Human Development, 68*, 83–91. http://dx.doi.org/10.1016/S0378-3782(02)00014-2

Knitzer, J. (2002). *Promoting social and emotional readiness for school: Toward a policy agenda. Set for success: Building a strong foundation for school readiness based on the social-emotional development of young children.* Kansas City, MO: Kaufman Early Education Exchange.

Knox, S. (2008). Development and current use of the Knox Preschool Play Scale. In L. Parham & L. Fazio (Eds.), *Play in occupational therapy for children* (pp. 55–70). St. Louis, MO: Mosby.

Kodak, T., & Piazza, C. C. (2008). Assessment and behavioral treatment of feeding and sleeping disorders in children with autism spectrum disorders. *Child and Adolescent Psychiatric Clinics of North America, 17*, 887–905, x–xi.

Korsten, J., Dunn, D., Foss, T., & Francke, M. (1993). *Every move counts: Sensory-based communication techniques complete kit.* Austin, TX: Pro-Ed.

Krakowiak, P., Goodlin-Jones, B., Hertz-Picciotto, I., Croen, L. A., & Hansen, R. L. (2008). Sleep problems in children with autism spectrum disorders, developmental delays, and typical development: A population-based study. *Journal of Sleep Research, 17*, 197–206.

Kroeger, K. A., Schultz, J. R., & Newsom, C. (2007). A comparison of two group-delivered social skills programs for young children with autism. *Journal of Autism and Developmental Disorders, 37*, 808–817. http://dx.doi.org/10.1007/s10803-006-0207-x

Lakes, K. D., Kettler, R., Schmidt, J., Haynes, M., Feeney-Kettler, K., Kampter, L., . . . Tamm, L. (2009). The CUIDAR early intervention parent training program for preschoolers at risk for behavioral disorders: An innovative practice for reducing disparities in access to service. *Journal of Early Intervention, 31*, 167–178. http://dx.doi.org/10.1177/1053815109331861

Lamm, N. C., De Felice, A., & Cargan, A. (2005). Effect of tactile stimulation on lingual motor function in pediatric lingual dysphagia. *Dysphagia, 20*, 311–324. http://dx.doi.org/10.1007/s00455-005-0060-7

Landa, R. J., Holman, K. C., O'Neill, A. H., & Stuart, E. A. (2011). Intervention targeting development of socially synchronous engagement in toddlers with autism spectrum disorder: A randomized controlled trial. *Journal of Child Psychology and Psychiatry, and Allied Disciplines, 52*, 13–21. http://dx.doi.org/10.1111/j.1469-7610.2010.02288.x

Larnert, G., & Ekberg, O. (1995). Positioning improves the oral and pharyngeal swallowing function in children with cerebral palsy. *Acta Paediatrica, 84*, 689–692. http://dx.doi.org/10.1111/j.1651-2227.1995.tb13730.x

Laud, R. B., Girolami, P. A., Boscoe, J. H., & Gulotta, C. S. (2009). Treatment outcomes for severe feeding problems in children with autism spectrum disorder. *Behavior Modification, 33*, 520–536. http://dx.doi.org/10.1177/0145445509346729

LaVesser, P., & Hilton, C. (2010). Self-care skills for children with an autism spectrum disorder. In H. M. Kuhaneck & R. Watling (Eds.), *Autism: A comprehensive occupational therapy approach* (3rd ed., pp. 427–468). Bethesda, MD: AOTA Press.

Law, M., Baptiste, S., Carswell, A., McColl, M., Polatajko, H., & Pollock, N. (2005). *Canadian Occupational Performance Measure* (4th ed.). Ottawa, Ontario: CAOT Publications.

Law, M. C., Cadman, D., Rosenbaum, P., Walter, S., Russell, D., & DeMatteo, C. (1991). Neurodevelopmental therapy and upper-extremity inhibitive casting for children with cerebral palsy. *Developmental Medicine and Child Neurology, 33,* 379–387. http://dx.doi.org/10.1111/j.1469-8749.1991.tb14897.x

Law, M. C., Darrah, J., Pollock, N., Wilson, B., Russell, D. J., Walter, S. D., . . . Galuppi, B. (2011). Focus on function: A cluster, randomized controlled trial comparing child- versus context-focused intervention for young children with cerebral palsy. *Developmental Medicine and Child Neurology, 53,* 621–629. http://dx.doi.org/10.1111/j.1469-8749.2011.03962.x

Law, M., Russell, D., Pollock, N., Rosenbaum, P., Walter, S., & King, G. (1997). A comparison of intensive neurodevelopmental therapy plus casting and a regular occupational therapy program for children with cerebral palsy. *Developmental Medicine and Child Neurology, 39,* 664–670. http://dx.doi.org/10.1111/j.1469-8749.1997.tb07360.x

Lekskulchai, R., & Cole, J. (2001). Effect of a developmental program on motor performance in infants born preterm. *Australian Journal of Physiotherapy, 47,* 169–176.

Lieberman, D., & Scheer, J. (2002). AOTA's evidence-based literature review project: An overview. *American Journal of Occupational Therapy, 56,* 344–349. http://dx.doi.org/10.5014/ajot.56.3.344

Limperopoulos, C., Bassan, H., Sullivan, N. R., Soul, J. S., Robertson, R. L., Jr., Moore, M., . . .

du Plessis, A. J. (2008). Positive screening for autism in ex-preterm infants: prevalence and risk factors. *Pediatrics, 121,* 758–765.

Linder, T. (2008). *Transdisciplinary Play-Based Assessment: A functional approach to working with young children* (2nd ed.). Baltimore: Paul H. Brookes.

Linscheid, T. R. (1992). Eating problems in children. In C. E. Walker & M. C. Roberts (Eds.), *Handbook of clinical child psychology* (2nd ed., pp. 451–473). New York: Wiley.

Losardo, A., & Notari-Syverson, A. (2001). *Alternative approaches to assessing young children.* Baltimore: Paul H. Brookes.

Love, J. M., Kisker, E. E., Ross, C., Raikes, H., Constantine, J., Boller, K., . . . Vogel, C. (2005). The effectiveness of Early Head Start for 3-year-old children and their parents: Lessons for policy and programs. *Developmental Psychology, 41,* 885–901. http://dx.doi.org/10.1037/0012-1649.41.6.885

Luiselli, J. K., O'Malley-Cannon, B., Ellis, J. T., & Sisson, R. W. (2000). Home-based behavior intervention for young children with autism/pervasive developmental disorder: A preliminary evaluation of outcome in relation to child age and intensity of service delivery. *Autism, 4,* 426–438. http://dx.doi.org/10.1177/1362361300004004007

Macy, M., Bricker, D., & Squires, J. (2005). Validity and reliability of a curriculum-based assessment approach to determine eligibility for Part C services. *Journal of Early Intervention, 28,* 1–16.

Maguire, C. M., Walther, F. J., van Zwieten, P. H., Le Cessie, S., Wit, J. M., & Veen, S. (2009). Follow-up outcomes at 1 and 2 years of infants born less than 32 weeks after Newborn Individualized Developmental Care and Assessment

Program. *Pediatrics, 123,* 1081–1087. http://dx.doi.org/10.1542/peds.2008-1950

Mahoney, G., & Perales, F. (2003). Using relationship-focused intervention to enhance the social–emotional functioning of young children with autism spectrum disorder. *Topics in Early Childhood Special Education, 23,* 74–86. http://dx.doi.org/10.1177/02711214030230020301

Mahoney, G., & Perales, F. (2005). Relationship-focused early intervention with children with pervasive developmental disorders and other disabilities: A comparative study. *Journal of Developmental and Behavioral Pediatrics, 26,* 77–85. http://dx.doi.org/10.1097/00004703-200504000-00002

Mandich, A., Polatajko, H., Miller, L., & Baum, C. (2004). *Paediatric Activity Card Sort.* Ottawa, Ontario: CAOT Publications.

Manikam, R., & Perman, J. A. (2000). Pediatric feeding disorders. *Journal of Clinical Gastroenterology, 30,* 34–46.

Marsden, D., Dombro, A., & Dichtelmiller, M. L. (2003). *The Ounce Scale User's Guide.* New York: Pearson Early Learning.

Martin, N. (2006). *Test of Visual–Perceptual Skills–3.* Los Angeles: Western Psychological Services.

Martin, N. (2010). *Test of Visual–Motor Skills–3.* Novato, CA: Academic Therapy Publications.

May-Benson, T. (2010). Play and praxis in children with an ASD. In H. Miller-Kuhaneck & R. Watling (Eds.), *Autism: A comprehensive occupational therapy approach* (3rd ed., pp. 383–426). Bethesda, MD: AOTA Press.

Mayo, N. E. (1991). The effect of physical therapy for children with motor delay and cerebral palsy: A randomized clinical trial. *American Journal of Physical Medicine and Rehabilitation, 70,* 258–267. http://dx.doi.org/10.1097/00002060-199110000-00006

McCart, A., Wolf, N., Sweeney, H. M., & Chai, J. H. (2009). The application of a family-based multi-tiered system of support. *NHSA Dialog: A Research-to-Practice Journal for the Early Childhood Field, 12,* 122–132. http://dx.doi.org/10.1080/15240750902774692

McConaughy, S. H., & Ritter, D. R. (2008). Best practices in multimethod assessment of emotional and behavioral disorders. In A. Thomas & A. J. Grimes (Eds.), *Best practices in school psychology V* (Vol. 2, pp. 697–720). Bethesda, MD: National Association of School Psychologists.

McCormick, M. C., Brooks-Gunn, J., Buka, S. L., Goldman, J., Yu, J., Salganik, M., . . . Casey, P. H. (2006). Early intervention in low birth weight premature infants: Results at 18 years of age for the Infant Health and Development Program. *Pediatrics, 117,* 771–780. http://dx.doi.org/10.1542/peds.2005-1316

McLean, M. (2005). Using curriculum-based assessment to determine eligibility: Time for a paradigm shift. *Journal of Early Intervention, 28,* 23–27.

McLean, M., & Crais, E. (2004). Procedural considerations in assessing infants and preschoolers with disabilities. In M. McLean, M. Wolery, & D. Bailey (Eds.), *Assessing infants and preschoolers with special needs* (pp. 45–70). Columbus, OH: Prentice Hall.

McManus, B. M., & Kotelchuck, M. (2007). The effect of aquatic therapy on functional mobility of infants and toddlers in early intervention. *Pediatric Physical Therapy, 19,* 275–282. http://dx.doi.org/10.1097/PEP.0b013e3181575190

McWilliam, R. (1991). *Children's Engagement Questionnaire.* Nashville, TN: Vanderbilt Center for Child Development.

McWilliam, R. (2010). *Routines-based early intervention: Supporting young children and their families.* Baltimore: Paul H. Brookes.

Melnyk, B. M., Alpert-Gillis, L., Feinstein, N. F., Fairbanks, E., Schultz-Czarniak, J., Hust, D., . . . Sinkin, R. A. (2001). Improving cognitive development of low-birth-weight premature infants with the COPE program: A pilot study of the benefit of early NICU intervention with mothers. *Research in Nursing and Health, 24,* 373–389. http://dx.doi.org/10.1002/nur.1038

Miller, L. J. (1988). *Miller Assessment for Preschoolers.* San Antonio, TX: Psychological Corporation.

Miller, L. J. (2006). *Miller Function and Participation Scales.* San Antonio, TX: Psychological Corporation.

Miller Kuhaneck, H., Henry, D., & Glennon, T. (2010). *Sensory Processing Measure–Preschool.* Torrance, CA: Western Psychological Services.

Moes, D. R., & Frea, W. D. (2002). Contextualized behavioral support in early intervention for children with autism and their families. *Journal of Autism and Developmental Disorders, 32,* 519–533. http://dx.doi.org/10.1023/A:1021298729297

Montgomery, P., Bjornstad, G. J., & Dennis, J. A. (2009). Media-based behavioural treatments for behavioral disorders in children. *Cochrane Database of Systematic Reviews, 2001,* CD002206.

Moore, E. R., Anderson, G. C., & Bergman, N. (2007). Early skin-to-skin contact for mothers and their healthy newborn infants. *Cochrane Database of Systematic Reviews 2007,* Issue 3, Art. No.: CD003519.

Morris, S., & Klein, M. (2000). *Pre-feeding skills: A comprehensive resource for mealtime development.* San Antonio, TX: Psychological Corporation.

Moyers, P., & Dale, L. (2007). *The guide to occupational therapy practice* (2nd ed.). Bethesda, MD: AOTA Press.

Mullen, E. M. (1995). *Mullen Scales of Early Learning.* Circle Pines, MN: American Guidance Service.

Mulligan, S. E. (2003). *Occupational therapy evaluation for children.* Philadelphia: Lippincott Williams & Wilkins.

Munakata, M., Kobayashi, K., Niisato-Nezu, J., Tanaka, S., Kakisaka, Y., Ebihara, T., . . . Onuma, A. (2008). Olfactory stimulation using black pepper oil facilitates oral feeding in pediatric patients receiving long-term enteral nutrition. *Tohoku Journal of Experimental Medicine, 214,* 327–332.

National Early Childhood Technical Assistance Center. (2012). *Annual appropriations and number of children served under Part C of IDEA.* Retrieved from http://www.nectac.org/partc/partcdata.asp

Neisworth, J., & Bagnato, S. (2004). The mismeasure of young children: The authentic assessment alternative. *Infants and Young Children, 17,* 198–212.

Nelson, M. N., White-Traut, R. C., Vasan, U., Silvestri, J., Comiskey, E., Meleedy-Rey, P., . . . Patel, M. (2001). One-year outcome of auditory–tactile–visual–vestibular intervention in the neonatal intensive care unit: Effects of severe prematurity and central nervous system injury. *Journal of Child Neurology, 16,* 493–498.

Newborg, J. (2004). *Battelle Developmental Inventory (2nd ed.) manual.* Rolling Meadows, IL: Riverside.

No Child Left Behind Act of 2001, Pub. L. 107–110, 116 Stat. 3071.

Office of Special Education Programs. (2010). *Data accountability center: Data tables for OSEP state reported data, Table 1-14*. Retrieved from https://www.ideadata.org/arc_toc12.asp#partbCC

Olafsen, K. S., Rønning, J. A., Kaaresen, P. I., Ulvund, S. E., Handegård, B. H., & Dahl, L. B. (2006). Joint attention in term and preterm infants at 12 months corrected age: The significance of gender and intervention based on a randomized controlled trial. *Infant Behavior and Development, 29,* 554–563. http://dx.doi.org/10.1016/j.infbeh.2006.07.004

Orton, J., Spittle, A., Doyle, L., Anderson, P., & Boyd, R. (2009). Do early intervention programmes improve cognitive and motor outcomes for preterm infants after discharge? A systematic review. *Developmental Medicine and Child Neurology, 51,* 851–859. http://dx.doi.org/10.1111/j.1469-8749.2009.03414.x

Parham, L., & Ecker, C. (2007). *Sensory Processing Measure (SPM): Home form.* Los Angeles: Western Psychological Services.

Parks, S. (1992–2006). *Inside HELP—Administration and reference guide.* Palo Alto, CA: VORT Corp.

Peacock, G., Amendah, D., Ouyang, L., & Grosse, S. D. (2012). Autism spectrum disorders and health care expecditures: The effects of co-occurring conditions. *Journal of Devopmental and Behavioral Pediatrics, 33*(1), 2–8.

Pinelli, J., Atkinson, S. A., & Saigal, S. (2001). Randomized trial of breastfeeding support in very low-birth-weight infants. *Archives of Pediatrics and Adolescent Medicine, 155,* 548–553.

Pinelli, J., & Symington, A. J. (2005). Non-nutritive sucking for promoting physiologic stability and nutrition in preterm infants. *Cochrane Database of Systematic Reviews, 2005,* CD001071. http://dx.doi.org/10.1002/14651858.CD001071.

Pletcher, L., & McBride, S. (2000). *Family-centered services: Guiding principles and practices for delivery of family-centered services.* Des Moines: Iowa Departments of Education, Human Services and Public Health. (www.extension.iastate.edu/culture/files/FamlCntrdSrvc.pdf)

Polichino, J., Clark, G. F., Swinth, Y., & Muhlenhaupt, M. (2007). Evaluating occupational performance in schools and early childhood settings. In L. Jackson (Ed.), *Occupational therapy services for children and youth under the IDEA* (3rd ed., pp. 23–58). Bethesda, MD: AOTA Press.

Poore, M., Zimmerman, E., Barlow, S. M., Wang, J., & Gu, F. (2008). Patterned orocutaneous therapy improves sucking and oral feeding in preterm infants. *Acta Paediatrica, 97,* 920–927. http://dx.doi.org/10.1111/j.1651-2227.2008.00825.x

Pridham, K., Brown, R., Clark, R., Limbo, R. K., Schroeder, M., Henriques, J., & Bohne, E. (2005). Effect of guided participation on feeding competencies of mothers and their premature infants. *Research in Nursing and Health, 28,* 252–267. http://dx.doi.org/10.1002/nur.20073

Punwar, A., & Peloquin, S. (2000). *Occupational therapy principles and practice* (3rd ed.). Philadelphia: Lippincottt Williams & Wilkins.

Rauh, V. A., Achenbach, T. M., Nurcombe, B., Howell, C. T., & Teti, D. M. (1988). Minimizing adverse effects of low birthweight: Four-year results of an early intervention. *Child Development, 59,* 544–553.

Reddihough, D. S., King, J., Coleman, G., & Catanese, T. (1998). Efficacy of programmes based on conductive education for young children with cerebral palsy. *Developmental Medicine and Child Neurology, 40,* 763–770. http://dx.doi.org/10.1111/j.1469-8749.1998.tb12345.x

Rehabilitation Act Amendments of 1973, §504 (amend, 29 U.S.C. §794).

Reichow, B., & Volkmar, F. R. (2010). Social skills interventions for individuals with autism: Evaluation for evidence-based practices within a best evidence synthesis framework. *Journal of Autism and Developmental Disorders, 40,* 149–166. http://dx.doi.org/10.1007/s10803-009-0842-0

Reid, J. (2004). A review of feeding interventions for infants with cleft palate. *Cleft Palate-Craniofacial Journal, 41,* 268–278. http://dx.doi.org/10.1597/02-148.1

Resnick, M. B., Armstrong, S., & Carter, R. L. (1988). Developmental intervention program for high-risk premature infants: Effects on development and parent–infant interactions. *Journal of Developmental and Behavioral Pediatrics, 9,* 73–78. http://dx.doi.org/10.1097/00004703-198804000-00004

Reynolds, C., & Kamphaus, R. (2006). *BASC-2: Behavior Assessment System for Children* (2nd ed.). Upper Saddle River, NJ: Pearson Education.

Robins, D., Fein, D., & Barton, M. (1999). *The Modified Checklist for Autism in Toddlers.* Storrs: University of Connecticut.

Rocha, A. D., Moreira, M. E., Pimenta, H. P., Ramos, J. R., & Lucena, S. L. (2007). A randomized study of the efficacy of sensory–motor–oral stimulation and non-nutritive sucking in very low birthweight infant. *Early Human Development, 83,* 385–388. http://dx.doi.org/10.1016/j.earlhumdev.2006.08.003

Romer, E. F., & Umbreit, J. (1998). The effects of family-centered service coordination: A social validity study. *Journal of Early Intervention, 21,* 95–110. http://dx.doi.org/10.1177/105381519802100202

Rush, D., & Shelden, M. (2011). *The early childhood coaching handbook.* Baltimore: Paul H. Brookes.

Russell, D., Rosenbaum, P., Avery, L., & Lane, M. (2002). *Gross Motor Function Measure (GMFM-66 and GMFM-88) user's manual.* London: Mac Keith Press.

Sackett, D. L., Rosenberg, W. M., Muir Gray, J. A., Haynes, R. B., & Richardson, W. S. (1996). Evidence-based medicine: What it is and what it isn't. *British Medical Journal, 312,* 71–72.

Sakzewski, L., Ziviani, J., & Boyd, R. (2009). Systematic review and meta-analysis of therapeutic management of upper-limb dysfunction in children with congenital hemiplegia. *Pediatrics, 123,* e1111–e1122. http://dx.doi.org/10.1542/peds.2008-3335

Sandall, S., Hemmeter, M. L., Smith, B., & McLean, M. (2005). *DEC recommended practices: A comprehensive guide for practical application in early intervention/early childhood special education.* Missoula, MT: Division of Early Childhood.

Schädler, G., Suss-Burghart, H., Toschke, A. M., von Voss, H., & von Kries, R. (2007). Feeding disorders in ex-prematures: Causes–response to therapy—Long term outcome. *European Journal of Pediatrics, 166,* 803–808. http://dx.doi.org/10.1007/s00431-006-0322-x

Schendel, D., & Bhasin, T. K. (2008). Birth weight and gestational age characteristics of children with autism, including a comparison with other developmental disabilities. *Pediatrics, 121,* 1155–1164.

Schultz-Krohn, W. & Cara, E. (2000). Occupational therapy in early intervention: Applying concepts from infant mental health. *American Journal of Occupational Therapy, 54,* 550–554. http://dx.doi.org/10.5014/ajot.54.5.550

Shelton, T., & Stepanek, J. (1994). *Family-centered care for children needing specialized health and developmental services.* Bethesda, MD: Association for the Care of Children's Health.

Shepherd, J. (2001). Self-care and adaptations for independent living. In J. Case-Smith (Ed.), *Occupational therapy for children* (pp. 489–527). St. Louis, MO: Mosby.

Shepherd, J. (2012). Self-care: A primary occupation. In S. Lane & A. Bundy (Eds.), *Kids can be kids: A childhood occupations approach* (pp. 125–157). Philadelphia: F. A. Davis.

Shonkoff, J., & Phillips, D. (2000). *From Neurons to neighborhoods: The science of early childhood development.* Washington, DC: National Academies Press.

Simpson, C., Schanler, R. J., & Lau, C. (2002). Early introduction of oral feeding in preterm infants. *Pediatrics, 110,* 517–522. http://dx.doi.org/10.1542/peds.110.3.517

Skard, G., & Bundy, A. (2008). Test of Playfulness. In L. D. Parham & L. Fazio (Eds.), *Play in occupational therapy for children* (2nd ed., pp. 71–94). St. Louis, MO: Elsevier/Mosby.

Social Security Act of 1965, Pub. L. 89-97, 79 Stat. 286, Title XIX.

Spagnola, M., & Fiese, B. (2007). Family routines and rituals: A context for development in the lives of young children. *Infants and Young Children, 20,* 284–299.

Sparrow, S., Cicchetti, D., & Balla, D. (2005). *Vineland Adaptive Behavior Scales* (2nd ed.). San Antonio, TX: Pearson.

Squires, J., & Bricker, D. (2009). *Ages and Stages Questionnaires* (3rd ed.). Baltimore: Paul H. Brookes.

Squires, J., Bricker, D., & Twombly, E. (2002). *Ages and Stages Questionnaires: Social–Emotional* (3rd ed.). Baltimore: Paul H. Brookes.

Stewart, K. (2010). Purposes, processes, and methods of evaluation. In J. Case-Smith & J. Clifford O'Brien (Eds.), *Occupational therapy for children* (6th ed., pp. 193–215). Maryland Heights, MO: Mosby.

Swick, K. J., & Williams, R. D. (2006). An analysis of Bronfenbrenner's bio-ecological perspective for early childhood educators: Implications for working with families experiencing stress. *Early Childhood Education Journal, 33*(5), 371–378

Tanta, K. J., Deitz, J. C., White, O., & Billingsley, F. (2005). The effects of peer-play level on initiations and responses of preschool children with delayed play skills. *American Journal of Occupational Therapy, 59,* 437–445. http://dx.doi.org/10.5014/ajot.59.4.437

Taub, E., Ramey, S. L., DeLuca, S., & Echols, K. (2004). Efficacy of constraint-induced movement therapy for children with cerebral palsy with asymmetric motor impairment. *Pediatric, 113,* 305–312. http://dx.doi.org/10.1542/peds.113.2.305

Teaford, P., Wheat, J., & Baker, T. (2010). *HELP 3-6 Assessment manual.* Palo Alto, CA: VORT Corp.

Tessier, R., Cristo, M. B., Velez, S., Giron, M., Nadeau, L., de Calume, Z. F., . . . Charpak, N. (2003). Kangaroo mother care: A method for protecting high-risk low-birth-weight and premature infants against developmental delay. *Infant Behavior and Development, 26,* 384–397. http://dx.doi.org/10.1016/S0163-6383(03)00037-7

Trombly, C. A. (1995). Occupation: Purposefulness and meaningfulness as therapeutic mechanisms (1995 Eleanor Clarke Slagle Lecture). *American Journal of Occupational Therapy, 49,* 960–972. http://dx.doi.org/10.5014/ajot.49.10.960

Turnbull, A., Turnbull, R., Erwin, E., Soodak, L., & Shogren, K. (2011). *Families, professionals, and exceptionality: Positive outcomes through partnerships and trust.* Upper Saddle River, NJ: Pearson Education.

Ulrich, D. (2000). *Test of Gross Motor Development* (2nd ed.). Framingham, MA: TheraPro.

Uniform Data System for Medical Rehabilitation. (2003). *Functional Independence Measure for Children—WeeFIM II System.* Buffalo, NY: Author.

VanLeit, B., & Crowe, T. K. (2002). Outcomes of an occupational therapy program for mothers of children with disabilities: Impact on satisfaction with time use and occupational performance. *American Journal of Occupational Therapy, 56,* 402–410. http://dx.doi.org/10.5014/ajot.56.4.402

Vaughn, S., Kim, A.-H., Sloan, C. V., Hughes, M. T., Elbaum, B., & Sridhar, D. (2003). Social skills interventions for young children with disabilities: A synthesis of group design studies. *Remedial and Special Education, 24,* 2–15. http://dx.doi.org/10.1177/074193250302400101

Vismara, L. A., Colombi, C., & Rogers, S. J. (2009). Can one hour per week of therapy lead to lasting changes in young children with autism? *Autism, 13,* 93–115. http://dx.doi.org/10.1177/1362361307098516

von Knorring, A.-L., Söderberg, A., Austin, L., & Uvnäs-Moberg, K. (2008). Massage decreases aggression in preschool children: A long-term study. *Acta Paediatrica, 97,* 1265–1269. http://dx.doi.org/10.1111/j.1651-2227.2008.00919.x

Voress, J., & Maddox, T. (2013). *Developmental assessment of young children (2nd ed.) (DAYC).* San Antonio, TX: Pro-Ed.

Wang, Q. (2005, July). *Disability and American families: 2000* (Census 2000 Special Reports). Washington, DC: U.S. Department of Commerce.

Whalen, C., Schreibman, L., & Ingersoll, B. (2006). The collateral effects of joint attention training on social initiations, positive affect, imitation, and spontaneous speech for young children with autism. *Journal of Autism and Developmental Disorders, 36,* 655–664. http://dx.doi.org/10.1007/s10803-006-0108-z

Whitaker, P. (2002). Supporting families of preschool children with autism: What parents want and what helps. *Autism, 6,* 411–426. http://dx.doi.org/10.1177/1362361302006004007

White-Traut, R. C., Nelson, M. N., Silvestri, J. M., Vasan, U., Littau, S., Meleedy-Rey, P., . . . Patel, M. (2002). Effect of auditory, tactile, visual, and vestibular intervention on length of stay, alertness, and feeding progression in preterm infants. *Developmental Medicine and Child Neurology, 44,* 91–97. http://dx.doi.org/10.1017/S0012162201001736

Wilder, D. A., Normand, M., & Atwell, J. (2005). Noncontingent reinforcement as treatment for food refusal and associated self-injury. *Journal of Applied Behavior Analysis, 38,* 549–553. http://dx.doi.org/10.1901/jaba.2005.132-04

Williams, K. E., Riegel, K., Gibbons, B., & Field, D. G. (2007). Intensive behavioral treatment for severe feeding problems: A cost-effective alternative to tube feeding. *Journal of Developmental and Physical Disabilities, 19,* 227–235. http://dx.doi.org/10.1007/s10882-007-9051-y

Willis, J. K., Morello, A., Davie, A., Rice, J. C., & Bennett, J. T. (2002). Forced use treatment of childhood hemiparesis. *Pediatrics, 110,* 94–96. http://dx.doi.org/10.1542/peds.110.1.94

Wilson, L., Mott, D., & Batman, D. (2004). The asset-based context matrix: A tool for assessing children's learning opportunities and participation in natural environments. *Topics in Early Childhood Special Education, 24,* 110–120.

Winnicott, W. (1964). *The child, the family, and the outside world.* London: Penguin Press.

Wolfberg, P. (1995). Enhancing children's play (Appendix: Play Preference Inventory). In K. A. Quill (Ed.), *Teaching children with autism:*

Strategies to enhance communication and socialization (p. 217). Independence, KY: Thomson Delmar Learning.

Wong, C., Kasari, C., Freeman, S., & Paparella, R. (2007). The acquisition and generalization of joint attention and symbolic play skills in young children with autism. *Research and Practice for Persons With Severe Disabilities, 32,* 101–109.

World Health Organization. (2001). *International classification of functioning, disability and health.* Geneva: Author.

Yeargin-Allsopp, M., Rice, C., Karapurkar, T., Doernberg, N., Boyle, C., & Murphy, C. (2003). Prevalence of autism in a U.S. metropolitan area. *Journal of the American Medical Association, 289,* 49–55.

Zeitlin, S., Williamson, G., & Szczepanski, M. (1988). *Early Coping Inventory.* Bensenville, IL: Scholastic Testing Service.

Zero To Three (2010). *Social–emotional development birth to 12 months.* Washington DC: ZERO TO THREE. Retrieved from http://main .zerotothree.org/site/DocServer/socemot_-_012_-_par.pdf?docID=10761&AddInterest=1503&JServSessionIda004=bbnhvzuel1. app201c

Subject Index

Note: Page numbers in italics indicate figures, boxes, and tables.

NICU interventions, 45
NICU-to-Home interventions, 45
nonstandardized assessments, 16, *17*
norm-referenced assessments, 16, *17*
NTrainer System, 44

obesity, 8
occupation, use of term, 3
occupational performance, analysis of, 19–23
occupational profile, 5, 16–19, *18*
occupational therapists, educational programs for, 59–60
occupational therapy assistants, educational programs for, 60
oral stimulation programs, 44
oral–motor skills, 28
outcomes planning, 11–12, 39–40

parent training, 50
parent-directed interventions, 43–44
Peabody Developmental Motor Scales, 48
performance patterns
    assessments for, *21*
    evaluation of, 27, 30
performance skills
    assessments for, *20–21*
    evaluation of, 26–30, *27*
physiological-based interventions, 44
play, 24–25. *see also* areas of occupation
policy, implications for, 58
poverty, statistics, 7
practice, implications for, 51
praxis skills, 27–28, *27*
prematurity, 7–8
process, 5

referrals, 13
regulation of occupational therapy practice, 60
Rehabilitation Act (1973), *9*, 10
reimbursement, 39
relationship-based interventions, 41
research, implications for, 58
rest and sleep, 23–24. *see also* areas of occupation
routines, 49–50

search strategies, 66–69, *67*, *68*
Sensory Processing Measures, 29
Sensory Profile, 24
sensory–perceptual skills, 28–29
service delivery
    in early childhood, 48–50
    process of, *4*
    recommendations for, *55–56*, *57–58*
services
    funding sources, 9–10, *9*
    requests for, 13
    settings for, 10
settings for services, 10, 15–16, 49
skin-to-skin contact, 44
sleep, 23–24. *see also* areas of occupation
social participation, 25. *see also* areas of occupation
Social Security Act (1965), *9*
social skills, 30
Social Stories, 42
social–emotional development
    implications for, 51
    interventions for, 40–42
    recommendations for, *52–53*
standardized assessments, 16, *17*
summative evaluation, 37
systematic reviews, 66–69, *67*, *68*

team models, 12
Test of Playfulness, 24–25
therapeutic use of occupations and activities, 36
therapeutic use of self, 36
therapist-selected toys and objects, 42
touch-based intervention, 40–41
toys, 42
transdisciplinary team models, 12
transitions, 38

Vermont Intervention Program For Low Birth Weight Infants, 41
video modeling, 42
visual-motor interventions, 48

Citation Index

Tessier et al. (2003), 40, 41, 72

Trombly (1995), 5, 12

Turnbull, Turnbull, Erwin, Soodak, and Shogren (2011), 8, 11, 12, 15

VanLeit & Crowe (2002), 50, 125

Vaughn et al. (2003), *33*, 42, 51, 83

Vismara, Colombi, & Rogers (2009), 41, 51, 77

von Knorring et al. (2008), *33*, 40, 73

Wang (2005), 15

Whalen, Schreibman, & Ingersoll (2006), 41, 45, 46, 57, 58, 78, 114

Whitaker (2002), 50, 58, 126

White-Traut et al. (2002), *31*, 44, 98

Wilder et al. (2005), *32*, 43, 86

Williams et al. (2007), *31*, 43, 51, 87

Willis, Morello, Davie, Rice, & Bennett (2002), 47, 105

Winnicott (1964), 3

Wong, Kasari, Freeman, & Paparella (2007), 45, 57, 58, 115

Yeargin- Allsopp et al. (2003), 8